Coping with
Kidney Disease

Coping with Kidney Disease

*A 12-Step Treatment Program
to Help You Avoid Dialysis*

Mackenzie Walser, M.D.

with
Betsy Thorpe

and contributions by
Nga Hong Brereton, M.S., R.D., I.B.C.L.C.

WILEY

John Wiley & Sons, Inc.

Published by John Wiley & Sons, Inc., Hoboken, New Jersey
Published simultaneously in Canada

Design and production by Navta Associates, Inc.

Limit of Liability/Disclaimer of Warranty: The information contained in this book is
not intended to serve as a replacement for professional medical advice. Any use of the
information in this book is at the reader's discretion. The author and publisher specifically disclaim any and all liability arising directly or indirectly from the use or applica-
tion of any information contained in this book. A health care professional should be
consulted regarding your specific situation.

For general information about our other projects and services, please contact our Cus-
tomer Care Department within the United States at (800) 762-2974, outside the
United States at (317) 572-3993, or fax (317) 572-4002.

Wiley also publishes books in a variety of electronic formats. Some content that
appears in print may not be available in electronic books. For more information about
Wiley products, visit our web site at www.wiley.com.

Library of Congress Cataloging-in-Publication Data:
Walser, Mackenzie.
   Coping with kidney disease: a 12-step treatment program to help you avoid dialysis/
Mackenzie Walser, with Betsy Thorpe, and contributions by Nga Hong Brereton.
      p.cm.
Includes bibliographical references and index.
   ISBN 0-471-27423-2 (Paper)
   1. Kidneys. 2. Kidneys—Diseases—Prevention. I. Thorpe, Betsy. II.
Brereton, Nga Hong. III. Title.
   RC902 .W34 2004
   616.6'1—dc22
                                                                    2003021346
Printed in the United States of America
10 9 8

To my wife, Betsy

Contents

Acknowledgments

This work arose from my care of 200 adults with chronic kidney disease in the Clinical Research Center of Johns Hopkins Hospital since 1984. I have kept my own records on all of them, and a number of publications already have resulted from this experience. I am particularly indebted to Sylvia Hill for decades of collaboration in every aspect of the work. Without her it simply would not have happened. Capable assistance in the Clinical Research Center was provided by Shirley Barnes, Romila Capers, Gloria J. Jones, Mary Missouri, Flo Perry, Wesla T. Zeller and others and in the Department of Pharmacology by Mimi Guercio. Hong Brereton, my current dietitian, has made major contributions both to the book and to the care of these patients, as have the several dietitians who preceded her: Keena Andrews, Elizabeth Chandler, Gloria Elfert, Tiffany Hays, Millicent Kelly, Celide Koerner, Chris Kutchey, Sylvia McAdoo, Helen Mullan, Elizabeth Tomalis, Mary Ann Van Duyn, Jean Wagner, Lynne Ward, and others. Until radioisotope determinations of kidney function were replaced by creatinine measurements following cimetidine ingestion, Helen H. Drew and Joanna L. Guldan capably performed most of these radioisotopic determinations, under the direction of Dr. Norman D. LaFrance. The many patients that I have followed over the years cannot be acknowledged by name (though many of their case reports appear here under aliases), but their loyalty and support has been critical. Many of them were referred by Dr. Luis F. Gimenez and by the late Dr. Daniel G. Sapir, to both of whom I am very grateful.

As to writing the book, I am indebted to my agent, Ed Knappman, for starting the ball rolling. I am greatly indebted to Dr. Gary Calton for detailed advice on the book and also to Dr. Paul J. Scheel, Jr., Dr. John Deeken, and Braxton Mitchell. My editor-writer, Betsy Thorpe, and I spent nearly a year transforming a book for doctors (the only kind I know how to write) into one for consumers, and I thank her for her help. Elizabeth Zack, Lisa Considine, and Kim Nir at John Wiley & Sons made many helpful comments. Support for the care of these patients and for the writing of the book was provided by grants from the National Institutes of Health, from the estate of Colonel Walter G. Shaffer, and by gifts from other patients.

Introduction

Kidney disease is a huge, underrecognized and undertreated problem in the United States. In *Coping with Kidney Disease*, I hope to raise awareness about this disease among patients and their families and caregivers, and strongly advocate the benefits of predialysis care. The cornerstone of this treatment is a very-low-protein diet, which, as I have shown through my work with patients at Johns Hopkins University, can effectively delay or indefinitely postpone the need for dialysis in those with kidney failure. This diet, and many other effective treatments, will be explained and illustrated with patient histories throughout the book, such as this one:

Horace Lysenko, a 54-year-old self-employed art consultant, was referred to me four years ago with the following history: One year before, he had developed severe kidney failure caused by obstruction from an enlarged prostate. The prostate gland, which surrounds the urethra, frequently becomes enlarged in older men, obstructing the flow of urine from the bladder. Following surgical relief of the obstruction, his kidney function was only partially restored: Two-thirds of his kidneys had been destroyed by the increased back pressure from his bladder. His kidney function was measured at one-quarter of normal. He was placed on a very-low-protein diet, supplemented by essential amino acids—the treatment outlined in this book. In the ensuing five years, his kidney function has actually improved somewhat. Despite severe damage to his kidneys, he remains free of symptoms and may never go on dialysis.

The Scope of the Problem

Like Horace, millions of Americans have reduced kidney function (that is, kidney failure), and don't know it. At least 6 million people have an elevated blood level of creatinine, a likely sign of kidney failure. Among older people with diabetes or hypertension (which includes the majority of older people), 1 in 8 has kidney disease. Among noninstitutionalized adults in the U.S., 1 in 10 has either an abnormal amount of protein in their urine or reduced kidney function, or both. Americans of all ages have kidney failure, especially older people, blacks, and Native Americans.

The Lack of Effective Care

Kidney failure is often undertreated by doctors. Patients frequently are told to come back for care only when they are in such discomfort that they are ready for dialysis. Numerous articles have been published in medical journals reporting various means to slow the downhill course of kidney disease; even so, most patients never receive these treatments. Untreated kidney failure usually progresses to end-stage renal disease, at which point dialysis or transplantation becomes essential for survival. Every year some 60,000 people start dialysis in the U.S. But many people on dialysis don't feel well. In fact, dialysis is so grueling that, according to the official government report of the U.S. Renal Data System for 1999, "1 in 5 patients withdraws from dialysis before death." In other words, in effect they commit suicide. It should be noted, however, that death by withdrawal from dialysis is usually a "good death," meaning that suffering is minimized. But clearly it is best to avoid dialysis as long as possible.

The Solution

First, kidney failure has to be identified, and then, measures to treat it must be undertaken. The United States is shockingly deficient in both areas.

Symptoms of kidney failure don't appear until most of kidney function has already been lost. However, people at risk for kidney disease can check their own urine using simple tests, and get their physicians to check their blood for problems early on. If more at-risk people found out earlier that they had kidney disease, they could markedly improve their future health by taking effective steps immediately.

This book lets people know about the available and effective treatments (many of which can be done in their own home) that can slow the progression of kidney disease. By these means, people can delay dialysis or transplantation for as long as possible or even totally avoid either procedure.

The treatment I describe alleviates symptoms markedly. Appropriate care for kidney failure includes a very-low-protein diet, with supplements, as well as blood pressure control and specific therapies to regulate the metabolism of sodium, potassium calcium, phosphorus, and acid, and to correct anemia, high blood cholesterol, and high blood uric acid (which causes gout). Certain drugs are helpful and others are contraindicated. Transplantation, which has become more successful but is limited by the number of donors, may become more widely available; this book discusses how.

Note: This book does not discuss children with chronic kidney disease. As children are treated at Johns Hopkins exclusively by pediatricians, I have no experience caring for them.

Ella Johnson, a 49-year-old schoolteacher came to Johns Hopkins in 1994 for treatment. She suffered from polycystic kidney disease, an inherited kidney disease that consists of cysts in the kidneys. Her mother had also had polycystic kidney disease and had been treated here for several years. Ella also had high blood pressure and recurrent urinary tract infections. Her left kidney could easily be felt during a physical exam, and was therefore considerably enlarged. She was placed on a low-protein diet supplemented by essential amino acids. She also started fish oil capsules and gets regular exercise. During seven years of follow-up, her kidney failure has progressed very slowly. The rate of loss of her kidney filtration capacity, also known as glomerular filtration rate, is only 1.8 ml per minute per year, compared with an average rate of about 7 ml per minute per year in patients with polycystic kidney disease. At this rate, she will be well into her 70s before she needs dialysis or a transplant.

How to Use This Book

The book is written for a lay audience: patients, their families, and care-givers. Part I presents a primer on kidneys, explaining what happens when kidneys fail and some of the reasons that might have led to their failure. Once that is established, we then move on to what can be done to make life better for a kidney failure patient.

Part II deals with treatment of kidney failure in the predialysis stage, in twelve steps. Chapter 7 sets forth the low-protein diet in detail and contains lists of common foods in order of their protein-to-calorie ratio and their phosphorus-to-calorie ratio (not previously published); this is invaluable information for patients who want to follow the life-saving low-protein, low-phosphorus diet.

Part III deals with measuring the progression of kidney failure, dietary treatment of the nephrotic syndrome (a related condition), med-ications for people with kidney failure, when to opt for dialysis, trans-plantation, and several case histories. A list of resources, including books, web sites, and useful products follows, as does a discussion of government support for low-protein diets. Notes are supplied to identify the sources of the information provided, but may be too technical for many readers. A glossary defines unfamiliar terms.

How I Came to Write This Book

I have spent 45 years here at Johns Hopkins University on the full-time faculty in the departments of pharmacology and medicine. Over the past 30 years, my colleagues and I have studied and worked with adult patients suffering from kidney failure, in the hopes of treating them effectively to delay dialysis. Through my studies and those of others, I have become convinced that the best treatment for those suffering from kidney failure is a very-low-protein, supplemented diet, with careful monitoring of lifestyle and of blood pressure to keep kidney failure from progressing. I wrote this book to share with you this knowledge, and hope that you can use it to learn to live with your kidney disease.

Terms, Measures, and Abbreviations

equivalent	A quantity of a chemical substance equal to the number of grams that participate in a particular chemical reaction with one mole of reactant
ESRD	End-stage renal disease
mcg	Microgram (one millionth of a gram)
mean	The average of a number of observations
median	The value above which half of the observations fall, and below which the other half fall. The median and the mean of a series of observations may differ considerably if there are a few extremely high or extremely low values. The median is more useful for some purposes.
mg	Milligram (one thousandth of a gram)
microalbuminuria	An increase in urine protein too small to be detected by the usual clinical tools: specifically, between 30 and 200 mg/day.
milliequivalent	One thousandth of an equivalent
millimole	One thousandth of a mole
micromole	One millionth of a mole

M	A concentration of one mole per liter of solution
mM	A concentration of one millimole per liter of solution
mole	A quantity of a chemical substance equal to its molecular weight in grams
millimole	One thousandth of a mole
micromole	One millionth of a mole
uM	A concentration of one micromole per liter of solution
proteinuria	Urinary protein

PART I

Looking at the Disease of Kidney Failure

1

What Do Kidneys Do and What Happens When They Fail?

Before we look at what you can do when your kidneys start to fail, it's a good idea to review the basics on how the kidneys work in the body. With this knowledge, you will get a better understanding of why the kidneys are so important in the functioning of your body and the extent of the damage that can occur to your health if things do go wrong.

The two kidneys lie in the abdomen on the muscles of the back, near the waist, and are about 5 inches long. The urine formed from each kidney passes down a long tube called the ureter into the bladder, which can expand to contain and store urine. When urine is passed out of the body, it goes through a tube called the urethra (see Figure 1.1 on the following page).

Each kidney is made up of about 1 million units, called nephrons, which begin with a filter, comprising a tuft of capillaries (the tiniest blood vessels), called the glomerulus. At the glomerulus, liquid is derived from the blood plasma, comprising a solution from which most of the protein

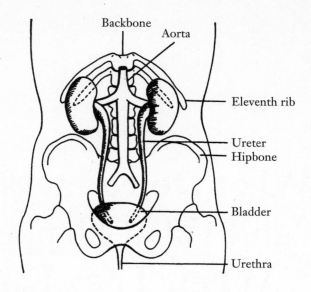

FIGURE 1.1: THE POSITION OF THE KIDNEYS.

From the kidneys, the ureters conduct urine to the bladder, which empties through the urethra. Blood is supplied to the kidneys by two renal arteries from the aorta, the main artery of the body. Reprinted by permission from *Kidney Failure, the Facts*, by Stewart Cameron, Oxford University Press, 1996.

has been filtered out by the glomerular membrane. This solution, called the glomerular filtrate, passes down a long, winding tubule (meaning little tube) and finally into a pouch called the kidney pelvis, which in turn drains into the ureter. During its passage down the tubule, most of the filtrate is reabsorbed, but some constituents are more completely reabsorbed than others; tubular secretion adds other constituents to the fluid. The final urine is small in volume compared to the glomerular filtrate, and differs from it considerably in composition.

By these multiple mechanisms the kidneys achieve their remarkable regulatory capacity. It is very important to recognize that the kidneys' main function is not to excrete wastes; instead, they play a very important role in keeping what is called extracellular fluid constant in its makeup. Extracellular fluid is the medium in which the millions of cells that make up our bodies are bathed. Blood plasma is part of the extracellular fluid, and it circulates throughout the body by the pumping of the heart. The kidneys keep constant the composition of the extracellular fluid, namely its content of salts, acid, nutrients, and many other constituents. The lungs play a similar role in that they remove carbon dioxide and add oxygen to the blood, so as to keep these two constituents constant.

The principal function of the kidneys is to keep constant the composition of the extracellular fluid, with respect to all other constituents. The kidneys also keep the volume of the extracellular fluid constant. By extraordinarily complex and efficient mechanisms, the kidneys regulate the excretion of water, salt, potassium, calcium, acid, and many other elements, whatever the intake of these substances may be.

Hormones regulate many of the kidney's functions. Hormones are like chemical messengers that are produced in other organs and sent to the kidney via the blood. For example, antidiuretic hormone, a hormone produced in the brain, is secreted in response to the concentration of dissolved solutes in body fluids. A high concentration of dissolved solutes, such as might occur after water loss in a hot environment, stimulates the production of this hormone. The kidney responds to the hormone by making the urine more concentrated and lower in volume, thus conserving water in the body. At the other extreme, a low concentration of dissolved substances, such as might occur after drinking a lot of water, turns off antidiuretic hormone production. As soon as the hormone disappears from the blood (about 30 minutes), the kidneys stop conserving water and do the opposite: The urine becomes very dilute and increases in flow, thus excreting the water load.

Urine flow can range widely depending on a person's intake of fluids: Minimal urine volume, during severe dehydration, may be as little as 250 ml a day (less than a pint), while maximum urine volume, in the absence of this antidiuretic hormone, is many gallons a day. People who can't make this hormone or who don't respond to it, because they have one form or another of a condition called diabetes insipidus (no relation to sugar diabetes), excrete huge volumes of urine and as a result get thirsty. Their fluid intake usually keeps up with their urine output, and they remain only slightly dehydrated most of the time.

The regulation of salt excretion is closely related to the regulation of body water because salt is the dominant dissolved substance in the extracellular fluid. Salt excretion is regulated by hormones that are produced by the adrenal cortex and by the heart. The regulation of salt balance is discussed in Chapter 8.

Another function of the kidneys is the production of important hormones, including:

- Angiotensin, a hormone that raises blood pressure by constricting blood vessels and also stimulates the adrenal cortex to produce yet another hormone, aldosterone, an important regulator of sodium excretion

- Erythropoietin, a hormone that stimulates the bone marrow to produce more red cells whenever their number is reduced; again, this explains why anemia is such a common feature of kidney failure

- Prostaglandins, which help regulate blood pressure, sodium excretion, and other functions.

In addition, the body's production of vitamin D takes place, in part, in the kidneys, which explains why vitamin D deficiency is a prominent feature of kidney failure.

Clearly, the kidney has many functions besides the excretion of wastes. You cannot live without your kidneys because of the important role they play. Complete loss of kidney function causes death within a few weeks. The good news is that we seem to have much more kidney function than we need, because with adequate care a person can survive with as little as 5 percent of normal kidney function. Thus donation of one kidney does not cause any signs of kidney dysfunction in the donor.

What Is Kidney Failure?

Kidney failure means loss of some (but not all) of the filtration capacity of the kidneys, which can be caused by a fall in blood pressure, a blockage of the blood circulation to the kidneys, blockage of urine outflow, or by disease of the kidneys themselves. Many different kinds of kidney disease are recognized, all of which cause loss of filtration capacity, but some of which are rapidly reversible. These reversible types of kidney failure are known as acute kidney failure.

Acute kidney failure can be caused by drugs toxic to the kidneys, by a severe reduction in kidney blood flow (for example, during surgery), and by many other causes. Urine output usually falls drastically, and waste products accumulate in the blood. But amazingly, complete recovery can occur within a few weeks. Patients often need dialysis temporarily.

Chronic kidney failure is generally not reversible, but often (though not always) gets progressively worse. When about two-thirds of filtration capacity is lost, symptoms of kidney failure begin to appear (see Chapter 3). When seven-eighths or so is lost, survival depends on either starting dialysis or transplanting a new kidney. This is called end-stage renal disease (ESRD).

How Big a Problem Is Kidney Failure?

Over 300,000 patients have end-stage renal disease and are currently on dialysis in the United States, and another 300,000 to 400,000 in other countries. (Hundreds of thousands of others who need dialysis in third world countries don't get it for economic reasons.) By 2010 there probably will be about 650,000 patients with ESRD in the United States, if the same rate of increase continues. Some of this increase represents wider availability; but kidney failure also seems to be getting more common.

These are the only statistics about the prevalence of kidney disease that have any reliability, and they do not measure prevalence of all cases of kidney failure; they measure the prevalence of end-stage kidney disease only, when dialysis is essential to survival. The prevalence of all cases of kidney disease in the United States can be estimated from large surveys of apparently normal samples of the population, in which a main indicator of kidney function, serum creatinine concentration, is measured in thousands of people. By determining what proportion of people in the sample has elevated creatinine levels and multiplying by an appropriate factor, we can estimate the prevalence nationwide.

The disturbing part of this equation is that most people with elevated serum creatinine levels are unaware of the fact. However, it is by no means certain that all of those who have elevated serum creatinine concentrations will go on to manifest chronic renal failure; in some, their serum creatinine level may spontaneously become normal; in others, it may remain slightly elevated but never rise further. For example, according to a recent study of 3,874 patients with elevated serum creatinine concentrations at an urban Veterans Administration center, followed for four years, many do not lose kidney function over time, including more than half of those with only slightly elevated levels and over a third of those with moderately severe kidney failure. It remains to be determined what differentiates those who progress to ESRD from those who do not.

In one large series of patients with chronic renal failure known as the Modification of Diet in Renal Disease Study, 15 percent exhibited no progression after being followed for at least two years. Sylvie Rottey and her colleagues in Belgium followed 83 patients with initial serum creatinine levels of 2 to 5 mg per dl for an average of five years. They found that half didn't progress at all during this interval.

The Diagnosis of Kidney Failure

How many people actually know they have chronic renal failure and have been properly diagnosed in order to receive treatment? Unfortunately, the answer to this question is not known even approximately. In a study reported at the American Society of Nephrology meeting in 2000, 889 U.S. relatives of dialysis patients were screened. The *majority* had signs of kidney disease, but most of these people were "unaware of their renal risk status." If we compare this statistic to people with diabetes, 70 percent of diabetics were aware that they had diabetes, while only 10 percent of subjects with evidence of chronic renal disease were aware of having it. Perhaps most alarming was the observation that the patients' physicians, when sent the results of the survey, often failed to change any aspect of their treatment. (We'll discuss this more in the next chapter.)

A survey of 1,436 adults in Venezuela revealed six individuals with persistently elevated creatinine levels, without apparent cause for acute renal failure. Only one of these six was aware of having chronic kidney disease. This was a surprisingly low frequency.

In a survey of 23,121 healthy Japanese schoolchildren, only 200 had signs of kidney disease, generally undiagnosed previously, emphasizing the relative infrequency of kidney disease in children.

In a large survey of apparently healthy adults in the United States, when the results were multiplied by the U.S. population, 800,000 adults nationwide were estimated to have serum creatinine levels above 2 mg per dl, and 10.9 million to have levels above normal (1.5 mg per dl).

Unfortunately, no surveys have determined how many of those surveyed were aware of having a high creatinine level. Defining prevalence in terms of measures whose results are not known to the subjects may be useful for fund-raising purposes, but it is not useful for these individuals' medical care.

A striking difference between true prevalence and diagnosed disease was shown in diabetic kidney disease by a report from Atlanta. In 1994 the authors reviewed hospital charts of 260 people with diabetes aged 64 to 75. Only 63 percent of the sample had their urine analyzed during their admission. Of these, 31 percent had urine protein of 1+ or greater, indicating advanced kidney disease. Twenty-five percent of the people with diabetes had elevated serum creatinine, but abnormal kidney function was noted in the discharge summaries of only 8 percent. "None [!] of these patients' medical records indicated that they had received dietary instructions about protein restriction, education about avoiding unnecessary use of NSAID's [nonsteroidal anti-inflammatory drugs, see Chapter 19], or education about diabetic renal disease." (These are some of the treatments we'll be discussing later in the book). Angiotensin-converting enzyme-inhibitors (ACEIs) or angiotensin-receptor blockers were no more likely to be used in those with abnormal renal function than in those without, despite the fact that these drugs are now widely recommended for patients with kidney disease (see Chapter 9). Thus most of these patients and their physicians apparently were unaware of the presence of renal disease and so did nothing about it.

A similar study of diabetic Medicare beneficiaries was reported from Seattle. Of 785 diabetics, 38 percent had urinary protein of 1+ or greater. But only 26 percent of patients known to have diabetic kidney disease and without contraindications to ACEIs were treated with ACEIs at discharge.

A recent report by Italian nephrologists documents similar findings. They reviewed the charts of 288 diabetics seen at a clinic in 1997. Although blood glucose was recorded in 99 percent, serum creatinine was recorded in only half and urine protein was seldom checked.

According to a recent summary, "30 percent to 40 percent of ESRD patients enter ESRD treatment only after an emergency-room visit triggered by undiagnosed renal failure." The authors conclude that "the pre-ESRD population is remarkably poorly followed."

In a recent review, the records of 155,076 patients who started dialysis between 1995 and 1997 were examined. Sixty percent of them had subnormal serum albumin concentrations, indicating malnutrition, and 51 percent had severe anemia. Only a small minority were treated by erythropoietin hormone injections, despite this drug being indicated for renal anemia (see Chapter 11). Heart disease was also prevalent and undertreated. The authors concluded that their data revealed "an alarmingly poor quality of pre-ESRD care among patients beginning dialysis in United States." Clearly this circumstance accounts in part for the high morbidity and mortality of ESRD patients in the United States. The authors were unable to explain the reasons for their findings.

One factor may be the official government attitude toward pre-dialysis care, which is well illustrated by a recent pamphlet for the general public entitled "Kidney Failure: Choosing a Treatment That's Right for You" released by the National Institute of Diabetes and Digestive and Kidney Diseases. The pamphlet describes dialysis and transplantation but makes no mention of predialysis care. However, the National Institutes of Health has started a program with the express purpose of education in predialysis care.

It is clear that early renal insufficiency is still widely ignored in the United States.

2

Are You at Risk for Kidney Failure?

Most people who have early kidney failure are unaware of their condition because of the notable lack of symptoms in the early stages. (We discuss symptoms in Chapter 3.) This is true in the case of other diseases too (like diabetes and hypertension) but is particularly common in kidney disease. So those people who are at risk for kidney failure, either because of inherited susceptibilities or risky behaviors, should be aware of the possibility of contracting a kidney problem. In Chapter 3 we discuss how easy it is to discover the presence of kidney disease by utilizing a simple at-home test, but first let's find out whether you fall into one of the at-risk groups.

Genetic or Family Predisposition for Kidney Failure

Men are slightly more susceptible to kidney failure than women. African Americans comprise 30 percent of those with end-stage kidney disease (ESRD), almost twice their frequency in the population at large. Native-born Americans and Pacific Islanders are also particularly susceptible, but anyone can get kidney disease.

The following groups of people are at high risk for developing kidney disease owing to inherited susceptibility.

Relatives of People on Dialysis

As mentioned, a majority of first-degree relatives of patients (siblings, children, and parents) with ESRD have signs of kidney disease and usually are unaware of it. The explanation is uncertain, but this observation suggests that congenital or familial factors may be of major importance. A check on urine protein and blood pressure of those at risk could identify most of those who may develop kidney failure. Such individuals need to check their own urine protein and their own blood pressure and report to their physician if either is abnormal.

Polycystic Kidney Disease

In this inherited condition, multiple cysts develop in the kidneys. On the average, half of the children of people with this disorder are destined to get the disease. About half of these, in turn, will develop kidney failure. Although all cases of polycystic kidney disease are the result of genetic defects, some of these are spontaneous mutations rather than inherited defects, so that not all patients will have an affected parent. DNA testing is available to determine the presence of the disease right from infancy, but is quite expensive, and the results can be confusing, because several genes may be defective. By age 20 or so, ultrasound examination of the kidneys can detect the disease. If it is present, multiple cysts will be found.

Without sophisticated tests, the disease may not become apparent until age 30 to 50. Sometimes the cysts become enormous, so that they are visible from outside the body. Protein in the urine is not always present during the early stages of the disease, so a blood test for creatinine may be required, followed by an ultrasound examination of the kidneys, to confirm the diagnosis.

Further complications with this disease sometimes include cysts in the liver, but they usually cause few ill effects. More serious are dilatations of the arteries in the brain (aneurysms), which can cause fatal bleeding, and should be surgically obliterated.

Some subjects at risk for polycystic kidney disease elect to forgo these tests and to rely on annual serum creatinine determinations, on the theory that, since no treatment is available, why get the bad news any sooner than you have to? This is obviously a difficult and complex choice, especially for people who plan to marry and have children.

There are also a number of inherited kidney diseases other than polycystic, although they are much less common.

Diseases That Lead to an Increased Risk of Kidney Failure

Sometimes it's the diseases you already have that can cause trouble for your kidneys. The most common culprits include diabetes and hypertension. A few patients develop kidney failure secondary to potassium deficiency.

Diabetes

People with either kind of diabetes (insulin-dependent and non–insulin-dependent) may get kidney failure after a decade or more of suffering from this disease. People with diabetes now comprise the largest group of patients starting dialysis in the United States and account for a large portion of the deaths from kidney failure. Diabetic kidney disease is relatively easy to detect in the early stages, because traces of protein appear in the urine. However, only one-third of subjects with traces of protein in their urine (microalbuminuria) will go on to develop full-blown kidney disease, with substantial amounts of protein in the urine. People with diabetes can and should test their urine for protein at least once a month. (Details of this test are given in Chapter 3.)

There is now evidence that close control of blood glucose levels in people with insulin-dependent diabetes somewhat reduces the incidence of kidney failure, though only at the cost of more frequent attacks of hypoglycemia. (see Chapter 16.)

For people with diabetes who are overweight (which many are), whether they are insulin-dependent or not, 20 percent weight loss, especially if combined with smoking cessation and increased exercise, can be extraordinarily beneficial. Not only does blood pressure decrease, but also the levels of blood fats (like cholesterol) fall; furthermore, in those who have kidney disease, kidney function improves and urinary protein loss diminishes. Thus all of the complications of diabetes are reduced.

Hypertension

High blood pressure is one of the most common disorders in the United States. The majority of people over 50 suffer from it. Thanks to a persistent campaign by the American Heart Association and others, the importance of controlling blood pressure is more and more widely known, and most patients now get at least some treatment for hypertension. Undertreated or untreated, hypertension can lead to heart failure, strokes, and kidney failure. It was widely assumed in the past that hypertension causes kidney failure.

However, a recent analysis of 10 large trials shows that controlling blood pressure in nonmalignant hypertension (the commonest kind) doesn't make any difference in the development of kidney failure. Among 26,521 people with high blood pressure followed for an average of five years, only 317 developed kidney failure. Patients who received antihypertensive drugs, who consequently had lower blood pressure than the others, did not have a significant reduction in their chances of getting kidney failure.

It is also widely held that African Americans are more susceptible than whites to kidney disease from hypertension. Dr. Norman Kaplan, an authority on high blood pressure, has recently summarized this issue, and concludes that it is true that most nondiabetic hypertensive African Americans with mild to moderate kidney failure have primarily hypertensive kidney disease. Yet only 10 percent of African Americans with kidney disease can be said to have hypertension as their primary disorder.

Thus the question as to just how often high blood pressure causes kidney failure remains unsettled, in contrast to the widespread view that it is a major cause. Whatever the case may be, it is still highly important for your overall health to treat hypertension effectively with the help of your doctor.

Pregnancy unquestionably makes hypertension worse. Consequently pregnant women should be closely monitored for the development or worsening of hypertension. Late in pregnancy, hypertension may be a sign of preeclampsia or eclampsia, serious complications. If you are pregnant, your blood pressure should be checked frequently.

Treatment of hypertension includes both lifestyle changes and drugs. Protein in the urine is an early sign of kidney damage from high blood pressure. Control of blood pressure is now known to be one of the most important features in the treatment of chronic kidney disease and may in fact stop progression altogether. But first kidney disease and hypertension have to be recognized.

Even in the absence of kidney disease, blood pressure should be maintained below 130/80, according to recent recommendations.

Potassium Deficiency

Potassium deficiency is another cause of kidney failure, though it is uncommon. Kidney function decreases in severe potassium deficiency and may never recover. Chronic diarrhea or overuse of laxatives can induce chronic potassium deficiency and renal failure. The ability of the kidneys to produce highly concentrated urine, and to decrease the output of urine in response to dehydration is characteristically impaired in patients with potassium deficiency, so these patients tend to excrete large volumes of urine (despite their reduced kidney function). Replenishing potassium stores usually restores kidney function, but not always.

Laura Melton came to Johns Hopkins at the age of 56. She told us that in order to lose weight, she had been taking laxatives every day for 30 years and still takes 2 to 3 pills daily. She had first exhibited urinary protein in an exam 11 years earlier. Three years before, she had 500 mg per day of urinary protein (normal urinary protein amounts to less than 150 mg per day) and a slightly elevated serum creatinine level (1.5 mg per dl; normal levels in women are below 1.3 mg per dl). Urinary protein had increased to 2.56 g per day. A kidney biopsy (removal of plug of kidney tissue with a needle) 10 months earlier showed glomerulosclerosis, meaning scarring of the glomeruli. Laura had had high blood pressure for three years, which had been treated irregularly. High serum cholesterol and triglyceride levels had been noted for at least 14 years, but had been treated only irregularly. Because of intermittent potassium deficiency, she was taking a potassium chloride supplement daily, but also taking a diuretic, hydrochlorothiazide, to lose weight. This diuretic causes increased potassium excretion (see Chapters 8 and 12), as well as increased salt excretion. Her physical exam was normal except for hypertension (160/100). Laboratory data showed mild renal insufficiency and serum potassium at the lower limit of normal. By the next visit, and for three years thereafter, while she showed up only occasionally, serum potassium was always subnormal, despite continuance of a potassium supplement. She admitted that she could not stop abusing laxatives, even at serious risk to her long-term health. At her last visit, after five years of follow-up, her renal failure had gotten only slightly worse. Subsequently she was lost to follow-up.

Laura's story illustrates how long-standing potassium deficiency (in this case self-induced) can cause kidney failure.

Glomerular Diseases

One of the most common causes of renal disease in my patients, as well as in the United States as a whole, is glomerular disease (glomerulonephritis or glomerulosclerosis). Glomerular diseases include a large list of disorders with varying causes, presentation, and predicted outcomes. These disorders can be treated with drugs, a discussion outside the scope of this book.

Behaviors and Medical History That May Lead to Kidney Failure

Chronic Use of Painkillers

Nonprescription analgesic drugs, sometimes called nonsteroidal anti-inflammatory drugs (NSAIDs), sold singly or in combinations, have the potential to cause kidney failure, when taken long term. Examples are Advil, Aleve, Alka-Seltzer, aspirin, BC Powder, Ecotrin, Excedrin, ibuprofen, Motrin, Tylenol, Vanquish, and many others. Combination drugs seem to be especially dangerous. NSAIDs are probably the most widely used drugs in the United States, but no one knows for sure how many patients with chronic kidney failure got there because of these drugs. If you must take medication for chronic pain, don't take it for more than a few days at a time.

Anyone taking these drugs for more than a week at a time should check their urine for protein at least once a month as described in Chapter 3. If there is protein in your urine, stop the drugs immediately and check again after a week or two. If protein persists, see your doctor. There is a group of patients whose renal disease is clearly caused by nonsteroidal inflammatory drugs. Analgesic abuse of this kind is much more common outside the United States (particularly in Switzerland and Australia). It follows years of near-daily ingestion of analgesics, usually two or more. Withdrawal of analgesics may reverse this kind of renal failure, but usually not if the failure is more advanced.

People Who Take Lithium Chronically

Lithium is widely used for the treatment of bipolar disorder. When it damages the kidneys (which it can do if the level of lithium in the blood gets too high), urine flow increases (sometimes to over a gallon a day). Protein may not appear in the urine at the early stages. Blood creatinine concentration will rise. Alternative medications, such as valproic acid, are available for the treatment of bipolar disorder, but may damage the liver.

Dieter Bacchus was an employee of city government. He developed bipolar disorder at the age of 21 and was started on lithium at age 24. His lithium and creatinine levels were checked regularly. By age 35, his serum creatinine concentration was noted as above normal, 1.8 mg per dl (normal is less than 1.5 mg per dl). By age 40, two glomerular filtration rate (GFR) determinations were 5.2 and 9.0 ml per min (normal is more than 100 ml per min). His lithium dosage was finally reduced, and by 1989 his GFR increased to 41.5 ml per min. He had no symptoms except that he had noted huge urinary volumes (8 liters a day) and also increased thirst. Urinalysis was negative.

He replaced lithium with valproate, which successfully controlled his manic episodes, but excessive water intake and large urinary volumes (6 to 8 liters daily) persisted. I advised him to start hydrochlorothiazde, a diuretic drug that, paradoxically, acts like antidiuretic hormone (weakly) and therefore reduces urine volume when the urine is very dilute, despite increasing salt excretion. He was not otherwise treated. Daily urine output decreased somewhat (to 4 to 6 liters per day).

Kidney function remained constant for five years. Then it began to decline, for unknown reasons, in association with an increase in average urinary protein excretion from 438 mg per day to 2,545 mg per day. Eventually his GFR fell to19.6 ml per min, and he was started on keto-conazole plus low-dose prednisone (see Chapter 16). A year later GFR was unchanged, indicating that the decline in GFR has been arrested. He has so far declined to follow a low-protein diet.

Dieter's story shows how excessive lithium administration can lead to kidney disease: At first his kidney function remained stable despite lithium, but eventually it has begun to decline. Switching to valproic acid from lithium stopped the kidney damage for a time. Starting ketocona-zole may have been a good move as far as the downhill course of his kid-ney failure is concerned. (See Chapter 16.)

Urinary Tract Obstruction

When the outflow of urine from the body is partially obstructed, either as the urine flows from the kidneys to the bladder or out from the blad-der via the urethra, back pressure may build up in the kidneys. This back pressure may distort the shape of the kidneys and diminish their function. This condition is called hydronephrosis. In some cases, complete urinary tract obstruction can develop and acute renal failure may occur. More commonly renal failure is only partial. By far the most common cause of urinary tract obstruction is enlargement of the prostate in men, but there are many other causes in women as well. When the obstruction is relieved, in most cases the kidneys have an amazing ability to recover from this damage, but the obstruction must first be recognized. A sono-gram of the kidneys and bladder will quickly reveal any obstruction. Surgery may be needed to relieve the obstruction. Urologists treat this type of kidney failure.

Corrective Surgery in Youth

Another urological problem arises in people whose childhood medical history includes difficulties with urinary drainage, especially reflux of urine from the bladder up the ureters into the kidneys during voiding. The multiple corrective operations that are needed may cause kidney failure. Mostly these patients are males. They may start to show signs of kidney disease in their 20s or earlier. It is best detected by measuring creatinine in the blood. Eventually they may progress to end-stage kidney failure.

Does Eating Too Much Protein Cause Kidney Failure?

One speculative cause of kidney failure is eating too much protein. The beneficial effect of protein restriction on the symptoms and the course of renal disease, discussed in Chapters 4 and 7, has logically led to the question as to whether a high intake of dietary protein can cause kidney disease. Some authors have gone so far as to recommend that older people in particular should cut down on dietary protein in order to reduce the incidence of kidney failure.

The evidence supporting the idea that high protein intake damages the kidney is unconvincing. The only experimental evidence supporting this idea comes from studies done on rats, especially after removal of one kidney and part of the other. Rats develop renal failure with age almost universally. (Many lab rats don't live long enough to get it.) The predominant lesion is a process called glomerulosclerosis. Although it was at first reported that protein intake was a determinant of this process, caloric intake was later shown to be just as important. Caloric restriction without protein restriction markedly retarded the development of glomerulosclerosis. Also, very high protein feeding for two years in rats had no effect on the extent of glomerulosclerosis.

Studies of this question in people have also cast doubt on the idea that protein harms normal kidneys. In a study of normal people, kidney function was measured in old individuals twice, separated by 10 to 18 years. A dietary history was taken from each person, and the protein content their diet contained was estimated. When the authors looked at the relationship between change in renal function over the 10- to 18-year interval and protein intake, they found no relationship. In other words, people who ate a lot of protein were just as likely to show a decline in kidney function with age as people who ate only a small amount of protein.

Other species do not exhibit the progressive decline in kidney function after partial removal of the kidneys that is characteristic of rats. Neither dogs nor baboons show this phenomenon, and they don't develop kidney damage from eating protein.

From these observations, it is clear that protein restriction does not prevent the decline in kidney function with age. In fact, reduced protein intake appears to be its major cause. A better way to prevent the decline with age would be to *increase* protein intake. Indeed, protein malnutrition in elderly people is a far more prevalent problem than is kidney insufficiency as a result of age-related decline in kidney function.

It seems safe to conclude that high dietary protein does not harm the kidneys in normal people.

Unknown Causes

There are many cases of kidney failure in which the cause is unknown. During the early stages of kidney failure, kidney biopsy can be performed to make a diagnosis, but not without some small risk. At later stages, kidney biopsy is more risky and should not be performed simply to clarify the diagnosis.

What Do You Do If
You Fall into a Risk Group?

If everyone in each of these categories got checked by measurement of urine protein, blood pressure, and blood creatinine level several times a year, most of the pre-dialysis patients in the United States would be identified. This would be a big step forward, and could lead to successful treatment in many cases. If you fall into one of these groups, read on.

3

Symptoms of Kidney Failure

Kidney failure, unlike disease of many other organs, does not lead to symptoms that point to the site of the problem. Pain in the kidney region, for example, is an unusual complaint, and contrary to what you might expect, patients with chronic kidney failure rarely note changes in urination. There is no change perceptible to the patient in the volume, color, appearance, or odor of the urine. Some persons with early renal insufficiency get up to urinate during the night more frequently, but this is by no means universal and has so many other causes that it cannot be considered a symptom of kidney impairment. While both the minimal volume of urine (during dehydration) and the maximal volume of urine (formed during water loading) are progressively reduced as kidney impairment becomes more severe, patients with chronic kidney failure almost never notice the change. Patients who develop the nephrotic syndrome (see Chapter 18) often notice foamy urine (due to its high protein content), whether they also have kidney failure or not. Although the symptoms of chronic renal failure are well known and are believed to be due to the biochemical abnormalities and the decrease in numbers of red cells in the blood (anemia) that characterize renal failure, there have been few attempts to relate these symptoms to specific abnormalities in a measured way.

Self-Testing

It is very easy to find out whether you have protein in your urine, which is an early sign of kidney disease. Protein in the urine can be detected simply by holding a paper strip (Uristrip and others) in the urinary stream. These strips are available without a prescription and can be found in or ordered by your local pharmacy. A change in color (see package insert) may indicate protein or glucose. If either is found repeatedly, tell your doctor. If you find that neither protein nor glucose is present your urine, you don't have to worry, but check frequently if you are in a high-risk group for kidney failure, for example, if you have diabetes.

What follows is a detailed discussion of the main symptoms of kidney failure. It is important to note, however, that none of these symptoms is common until most kidney function has been lost: The presymptomatic stage of kidney failure lasts many months to many years. If you already know that you suffer from kidney failure, and you didn't recognize the symptoms when they first appeared, don't beat yourself up over it. There's still more you can do. If you are at risk for getting kidney failure, it is more important to get tested in your doctor's office regularly than it is to watch for these symptoms.

Fatigue

The most common symptom of chronic kidney failure, and one of the earliest, is fatigue. This can take the form of a constant feeling of tiredness, lack of a sensation of well-being, lack of energy, tiredness at the end of the day, or fatiguability (that is, becoming tired quickly during even mild activity). These types of fatigue are to be distinguished from shortness of breath on exertion and also from muscle fatiguability, such as weakness of the legs on walking or climbing stairs. As you might expect, many people have difficulty distinguishing the subtle differences between these symptoms.

Doctors don't fully understand the cause of fatigue in patients with chronic kidney failure. In severely anemic patients it is caused by the anemia itself (see Chapter 11), but the degree of fatigue in most patients is clearly out of proportion to the severity of the anemia.

The point at which fatigue develops during the slow downhill course of chronic kidney failure is extraordinarily variable. I have seen patients complain of it when they still had most of their kidney function left, and others steadfastly deny fatigue despite a red blood cell count as low as 60 percent of normal and having lost nearly all of their kidney function. Part of these differences can be attributed to stoicism, at one extreme, and a tendency to exaggerate complaints at the other, but that doesn't account for all of it. Obviously fatigue is a very nonspecific complaint that may have many possible explanations.

Dietary treatment reduces fatigue but unfortunately doesn't usually eliminate it. This symptom remains one of the most prevalent causes of disability in chronic kidney failure. Better treatment of anemia (with ery-thropoietin, see Chapter 11) may reduce fatigue considerably.

Muscle Cramps

The second most common complaint of patients with chronic kidney failure is muscle cramps. Typically these cramps involve the calf muscles, but they can occur in any muscle group. Involuntary contraction of the involved muscle(s) occurs, often at night, and may be quite painful. Some patients never develop muscle cramps. This complaint isn't quite as nonspecific as fatigue, but certainly does occur in healthy individuals, particularly following strenuous use of a muscle that isn't called upon often.

Again, doctors do not know what causes muscle cramps in patients with kidney disease. Potassium depletion also can cause muscle cramps, and patients who require potassium supplements (see Chapter 12) often note that omitting these supplements makes cramps worse. But potassium depletion is not the cause of muscle cramps in most kidney patients. Salt depletion also can cause muscle cramps, but this is rarely the cause in patients with kidney disease.

For unknown reasons, dietary treatment regularly reduces or eliminates muscle cramps. Also, cramps often can be relieved by quinine sulfate (available without a prescription). A dose of 300 mg or less, either when cramps occur or as a preventive, for example, at bedtime, often helps. Quinine is far from safe. In substantial dosage, it can cause allergic reactions that deplete elements of the blood, with disastrous consequences. For example, a 64-year-old man recently developed a life-threatening bleeding disorder after taking 2 to 5 large bottles of tonic containing quinine daily for 2 to 3 weeks to ward off muscle cramps.

Loss of Appetite, Nausea and Vomiting

Loss of appetite, nausea, and vomiting are well-known symptoms of severe kidney failure. Typically they appear when the blood urea concentration gets quite high, but some changes in appetite, particularly an aversion to meat, may occur much earlier. Weight loss is uncommon early on. Our study, summarized in detail at the end of this chapter, suggests that anemia may be a significant factor in nausea and vomiting—unlikely though this seems. Dietary treatment, as outlined in Chapter 7, usually improves appetite.

Easy Bruising

Easy bruising is often noticed in patients with severe kidney failure, and sometimes in those with quite mild kidney failure. This symptom is hard to define, and many people will say that they have always bruised easily. But in severe cases, the forearms and hands may become mottled with bruises. Presumably this reflects the increased fragility of the capillaries. No treatment is known to be effective, although some drugs have been tried with questionable success.

Itching

Dry skin is characteristic of relatively severe kidney failure, but is not particularly distressing as a symptom. Itching, however, is a common and sometimes very distressing symptom. It doesn't usually appear until loss of kidney function is severe (about 80 percent). Its cause is also unknown. Our study, summarized at the end of the chapter, suggests that both acidosis and anemia can contribute to itching. Itching may be confined to the torso or may be all over. Dietary treatment regularly reduces it, but in my experience does not usually eliminate it. This same complaint is common in patients on dialysis and is thought to be correlated with the concentration of plasma phosphate. We could not substantiate this finding in predialysis patients, but the marked elevation of serum phosphate concentration often seen in this group was not seen in this group.

Treatment for dry and itching skin is not very helpful for patients with kidney failure. Moisturizing preparations may decrease the itching somewhat. Antihistamines have been used with variable results. In severe cases, ultraviolet light treatments can be tried.

Shortness of Breath on Exertion

Shortness of breath on exertion is not, strictly speaking, a symptom of kidney failure, but rather a reflection of one of its complications—either severe anemia or congestive heart failure, or both. The symptom is important, though, because it may indicate that treatment of the anemia or fluid retention is urgent.

Other Less Common Symptoms

Other symptoms of kidney failure include thirst, headache, a bad taste in the mouth, somnolence, insomnia, twitching or restless legs, difficulty concentrating, impaired memory, numbness and tingling in the hands and feet (reflecting nerve damage from uremia), voiding frequently at night (reflecting impaired urinary concentrating ability), diarrhea, and constipation.

Dependence of Symptoms
on Lab Results

Although the symptoms of chronic renal failure are well known and are believed to be the consequence of chemical abnormalities of the body fluids, there have been few attempts to relate these symptoms to specific abnormalities.

In an effort to see if symptoms can be correlated with lab results, Ramesh Mazhari and I conducted a study based on the symptoms of 167 patients with chronic kidney disease (renal failure or the nephrotic syndrome). They were graded as to the severity of the disease, based on their biochemical abnormalities, and the severity of their anemia. We chose four symptoms to analyze in detail: fatigue, muscle cramps, itching, and nausea and vomiting. When we placed most of these patients on dietary treatment, in many cases symptoms improved or disappeared. In the second analysis, we documented the level of each of the lab measurements we used to determine severity of kidney failure when, during follow-up and worsening of their renal failure, these same symptoms reappeared (or appeared for the first time). Thus we obtained two estimates of how these symptoms depend on the abnormalities seen in blood tests.

We were disappointed to find that none of the abnormalities in the tests predicted the common symptoms of kidney failure. The main conclusion from this study is that common blood test indicators cannot explain the symptoms of chronic renal failure.

In a similar study in a smaller number of patients, Birgitta Klang and Naomi Clyne found that the degree to which the body fluids had become abnormally acid, as indicated by how much the level of serum bicarbonate was reduced below normal, was correlated with both leg cramps and itching. This finding is of particular interest because the bicarbonate level was 18 mM or higher in their patients, and some laboratories consider such levels to be within normal limits. (see Chapter 10.)

Another surprise in our study was that nausea and vomiting were correlated only with hematocrit level; thus anemia seemed to be the strongest determinant of nausea and vomiting. Conventional wisdom would have predicted that the severity of renal failure, measured as serum urea or creatinine, or glomerular filtration rate, would have been the principal determinant of nausea and vomiting. Klang and Clyne, by contrast, found that nausea and vomiting were correlated with the concentration of albumin in the serum.

Perhaps most surprising in both studies was that serum levels of calcium, phosphate, and iron were not correlated with any of these symptoms, even though these levels often were often abnormal.

In the next chapter we'll take a look at ways of coping with kidney failure.

PART II

HOW TO TREAT KIDNEY FAILURE

4

Treating Kidney Failure

Until about 1970, kidney failure meant death. When the kidneys stop functioning, harmful wastes build up in the body, blood pressure rises, and excess fluid may be retained, sometimes causing heart failure. As discussed in Chapter 1, the kidneys perform so many complex functions that in the past it was difficult for the medical community to treat kidney failure. Now there are three ways to treat kidney failure: dialysis, transplantation, and diet. None of these choices, however, is an ideal solution.

To quote Dr. Robert Berliner, a mentor of mine:

It must be recognized . . . that dialysis and transplantation represent the epitome of what [Lewis] Thomas has dubbed "half-way technology"—methods, only modestly satisfactory, that place great demands on time and resources that are needed only because we are as yet unable to come to grips directly with the processes underlying the diseases that destroy the kidneys and make end-stage disease a reality to be dealt with. This burden will be reduced only when we have improved our understanding of the initiating factors in chronic renal disease and the nature of the processes that perpetuate the progressive damage and have learned how to prevent or interrupt them. The progress made in recent years in dissecting pathologic entities and in elucidating immunologic mechanisms offers encouragement that the day may be not far distant when the dialyzer, at least for chronic dialysis, will take its place with the iron lung.

Dr. Berliner wrote these words in 1976. More than 25 years later, the day has still not arrived, but at least there is hope, as this book documents.

Let's first take a look at dialysis.

Dialysis

How Dialysis Works

Back in 1912, the idea of an artificial kidney was conceived at Johns Hopkins School of Medicine in the Department of Pharmacology, where I now work. Dr. John Jacob Abel, the first head of this department, with Leonard Rowntree and Benjamin Turner, tested and then published their experience with an artificial kidney in dogs. The principle is quite simple, but the practice is not: The blood is exposed, through a membrane permeable to water and small molecules but not permeable to proteins, to a solution similar in composition to body fluids, but minus the products of protein breakdown that accumulate in the blood when the kidneys fail. These products diffuse across the membrane, reducing their level in blood and body fluids. Abel, Rowntree, and Turner intended to use this technique to remove drugs toxic to the kidney from patients' blood. Sometimes artificial kidney treatment is used for this purpose even now. But most of the time it is used to treat kidney failure.

During World War II a Dutch physician, Dr. Willem J. Kolff, and his associates first successfully used an artificial kidney, although the longest they succeeded in keeping someone alive with no kidney function was 26 days. Their patients had acute kidney failure, usually as a result of injuries.

In 1960 Dr. Belding Scribner and his associates in Seattle devised a method of access to the blood in the form of a shunt made of Teflon. Until then it had been necessary to use glass or metal connections, which soon clotted. Teflon made it possible for the first time to keep patients with end-stage renal disease alive. Scribner's team began treating outpatients repeatedly with dialysis for months and even years. The Teflon shunt has now been superseded by a direct connection between an artery and a vein, called an arteriovenous fistula, or by a graft, which connects an artery to a vein with a synthetic tube.

The peritoneum (the membrane that encloses the intestines and the other abdominal organs) is highly permeable. Dr. Arthur Grollman, at the Southwestern Medical of the University of Texas in Dallas, demonstrated in the 1950s that dogs whose kidneys have been removed could be kept alive by repeatedly injecting salt solution into the abdominal cavity and later removing it. Substances like urea and creatinine diffused from the blood across the peritoneal membrane into the fluid. Chronic peritoneal dialysis became practical only after Dr. Henry Tenckhoff developed a peritoneal catheter that could be used long term. Now this technique is as widely used as the original hemodialysis technique, and patients may be treated by either method.

Unless they have received a transplanted kidney, patients with end-stage kidney disease (ESRD) must get regular dialysis by either hemodialysis or peritoneal dialysis. Hemodialysis usually involves visits to a dialysis unit three times a week for several hours. Peritoneal dialysis usually involves running a large volume of fluid into the abdominal cavity by way of a permanently implanted tube and, after a few hours, draining it out and putting in more. This process is repeated more or less continuously. (For additional details about dialysis options, see Chapter 21.)

These two techniques are very different, and discussing their relative merits is a complex task. I recommend that those who are interested read *Treatment Methods for Kidney Failure: Hemodialysis* and *Treatment Methods for Kidney Failure: Peritoneal Dialysis*, both published by the National Institute of Diabetes and Digestive and Kidney Diseases.

Free Dialysis Care

Chronic kidney failure is the one and only disease whose treatment is almost completely paid for by the U.S. government. This unique situation is the result of the passage, in 1972, of legislation that authorized the End-Stage Renal Disease program. This program provides reimbursement for all of the costs of dialysis and/or transplantation to patients certified to be at the end stage, after two and one-half years during which they (or their insurers) must pay. Peritoneal dialysis was not covered initially, but in 1978 the Food and Drug Administration (FDA) approved continuous peritoneal dialysis for the treatment of ESRD. Medicare began reimbursing the costs in 1979.

The supporters of this legislation did not anticipate how the need for this treatment would grow. Today there are over 300,000 patients in the ESRD program in the United States, at an average annual cost per patient of $40,000, for a grand total of more than $12 billion per year. This figure excludes drug costs, which are substantial, especially for treatment of anemia.

The Problem with Dialysis

Dialysis is life-saving, and we are lucky to have it to extend the lives of those with kidney failure. The difficulty with this program, apart from its high cost, is that it is a far from ideal solution for most patients. Regular dialysis is an enormous physical burden. Many dialysis patients do not feel well and suffer from fatigue or sometimes more specific complaints, such as weakness, itching, muscle cramps, shortness of breath, and nausea. Only about half continue working; the others collect disability benefits.

The death rate of patients on dialysis in the United States is still alarmingly high, over 20 percent per year, although it has fallen steadily since 1988. Part of this high mortality is attributable to the fact that a significant number of new dialysis patients are near death from other causes. Most of these deaths are apparently from cardiovascular disease, but the proportion is difficult to pin down from the available government reports. The 1999 summary, entitled U.S. Renal Data System, stated that "1 out of 5 dialysis patients withdraws from dialysis before death." In other words, these patients voluntarily stopped treatment. This depressing cause of death has disappeared in the more recent summaries. Sad as it may seem, withdrawal from dialysis is reported to be a "good death," meaning that suffering is minimized.

Now that we have looked at dialysis, let's consider kidney transplants.

Kidney Transplants

Transplantation, if successful, is associated with a higher rate of rehabilitation and lower mortality than dialysis. But among the numerous problems with this treatment, the primary one is that there are too few donor kidneys compared to the number of people who need them. Recovery takes a long time. And to make sure you don't reject the transplant, you need continuous drug treatment (which has its own dangers) and close monitoring. We will discuss the details of transplantation in Chapter 20.

The Low-Protein Diet
(and Predialysis Treatment)

Before putting any patient on dialysis, doctors have an obligation to tell the patient that there is an alternative available, namely dietary treatment and close follow-up to watch for the other conditions that could endanger the patient with kidney failure. The low-protein diet is discussed in detail in Chapter 7, and other complications and their treatments are discussed in the following chapters. But let's explore the case for (and against) this alternative treatment that I advise as a first line of treatment.

The Argument for the Low-Protein Diet

Let me explain the benefits of the low-protein diet and predialysis care. We have reported that in 76 patients, a very-low-protein diet with a supplement of amino acids or ketoacids safely defers dialysis for an average of more than one year. Good nutrition was well maintained during this time, despite the low intake of protein. This is critical, because protein malnutrition at the start of dialysis bodes ill for survival.

A similar study was conducted by French researcher Michel Aparicio and colleagues. They treated 176 patients with the same diet and supplements and confirmed our results. In both studies, serum albumin level (an index of protein nutrition) was well maintained despite the low protein intake; subsequent mortality of these same patients on dialysis was not increased; on the contrary, it was surprisingly low. Three other studies confirm these findings.

By contrast, 60 percent of patients entering dialysis nationwide in the United States are malnourished, as shown by their subnormal serum albumin levels.

Since 1983 I have treated 129 patients with a supplemented very-low-protein diet. At the start of their diet, the patients' serum creatinine levels, which measure their level of kidney failure, averaged 4.2 mg per dl.

(The normal level is less than 1.5 mg per dl.) Despite this severe level of kidney failure, at least one-third of these patients have succeeded in deferring dialysis for over 40 months.

Compare this record with the data on the interval between diagnosis of renal failure and the start of dialysis in all the patients who started dialysis at Johns Hopkins and at Royal Victoria Hospital in Montreal over a period of seven years. Their average serum creatinine at the time of diagnosis was 4.7 mg per dl. By 10 months from diagnosis, with essentially no treatment, nearly half of them were on dialysis.

Why You May Not Have Heard about This Treatment

The existence of the ESRD program has led to an unfortunate lack of attention by nephrologists and by funding agencies to treatment of chronic kidney failure in the stages before dialysis. Sadly, while nephrologists and internists may recognize kidney failure, they may advise no treatment, telling patients to wait until they're symptomatic, at which point a funded treatment program is available for everyone. Doing this would make sense if the results of dialysis and transplantation were totally satisfactory, but they are far from it.

Some physicians ignore laboratory evidence that their patients have early kidney failure and fail to tell them, for example, which drugs might help, which drugs to avoid, or mention anything about the dangers of smoking or the benefits of nutritional approaches. In some amazing cases, year after year physicians fail to tell patients that they have kidney disease. Predialysis renal failure seems to be nearly unique in the extent to which it is neglected.

Even the experts tend to neglect the dangers of kidney disease. For example, the American Diabetes Association's book for patients, *Complete Guide to Diabetes*, does not mention self-tests for urine protein and devotes only four pages (out of 446) to kidney disease, even though this is a major problem for patients with diabetes.

Consumer Reports recently featured an article entitled "Taking Charge of Diabetes: Self-Care Is Crucial and Widely Neglected." Yet the article makes no mention of testing for urine protein and instead is devoted entirely to testing blood sugar.

Self-tests for serum creatinine or cystatin C level are not currently on the market, but either one could be devised easily.

One reason that few patients get any advice on treatment for predialysis kidney disease is that widespread skepticism exists regarding the value of this treatment. I'm not entirely sure why this is the case, but I have a strong suspicion that physicians like myself who work with predialysis patients may have oversold our approach to the point where other nephrologists have become increasingly skeptical. This skepticism is particularly prevalent among academic nephrologists, less so among practicing nephrologists and internists, many of whom try to achieve the same aims as are outlined in this book. It is also true that physicians in general are skeptical of dietary treatments, preferring to administer medications.

The use of a supplemented very-low-protein diet predialysis continues to be "controversial." Furthermore, some nephrologists, such as Gerald Schulman and Raymond Hakim, go so far as to state, "Protein intake [in predialysis patients] . . . should not be permitted to fall below 0.8 g/kg per day [56 g per day, in a 70 kg person]." On the contrary, Drs. Mitch, Maroni, Kopple and I believe all patients should have a trial of a protein-restricted diet before being placed on dialysis, as we pointed out in our editorial in the journal *Kidney International* in 1999. Many patients will exhibit striking improvement in symptoms, and the diet presents no risks.

Some of this skepticism can be attributed to our claims that predialysis treatment can slow the progression of chronic renal failure, a claim that has been difficult to document in a way that convinces everyone. Skepticism on this issue has led to an illogical disinterest in predialysis care. Even if progression cannot be slowed by diet, careful predialysis care is worthwhile.

It is essential to differentiate between two possible benefits from predialysis treatment: (1) slowing the rate at which kidney function fails, and (2) reducing symptoms at any given level of kidney impairment. The first remains somewhat controversial (although I am convinced of its validity), but the second has been unequivocally established for at least 100 years. If you think about it, you will realize that these two possible benefits are closely interrelated. Dialysis typically is begun when symptoms reach a certain level of severity. If symptoms can be reduced (without change in kidney function), dialysis can be deferred, at least for a few months.

A third and even more important aspect of predialysis treatment that has not been adequately emphasized is control of all those aspects of chronic kidney failure that not only can cause symptoms, but can cause premature and sudden loss of remaining kidney function or cause death in patients whose kidney function was still relatively well maintained before such complications occurred. In fact, many patients begin dialysis not because their kidney failure progressed to the end stage, but because one or more of the complications caused such severe symptoms that dialysis was the only obvious solution. Some of the more common complications that can precipitate dialysis are congestive heart failure caused by salt and water overload (Chapter 8), severe acidosis (Chapter 10), high serum potassium (Chapter 12), high serum calcium (Chapter 13), and the use of drugs that cause acute kidney damage (Chapter 19). Other complications, including hypertensive crisis and stroke (Chapter 9), can cause death long before the end stage is reached.

Careful attention to all of the many aspects of kidney failure in the predialysis stage will not only permit a nearly symptom-free existence up to the point that dialysis or (preferably) transplantation may become unavoidable (and will significantly postpone that point, perhaps indefinitely), but will also make it possible to avoid the large list of complications that may occur as kidney function gets worse.

Is Remission of Kidney Failure Possible?

There has been a lot of talk recently about "remission" of chronic renal failure. A decrease in the loss of protein in the urine, in the absence of kidney failure, or when the kidney disease is acute, certainly does occur. But a small scarred kidney is not going to grow back into a normal one, no matter what. There is no such thing as remission of chronic renal failure.

However, arresting the progression of the disease is a real possibility, as shown by a number of publications and by several detailed accounts of patients given in Chapter 22. If kidney failure can be arrested permanently before it gets severe enough to cause symptoms, the only problem for the patient is the drugs and/or diet that must be followed for this situation to continue. This is not remission, but arrested progression.

I did have one case of real remission (page 160), in which kidney function rose to normal. This must mean that the low kidney function seen at the patient's first visit was caused not by chronic renal failure but by profound changes in kidney blood flow. The patient probably never had a loss of functioning units in the kidney. The nephrotic syndrome (see Chapter 18) caused these changes in renal blood flow; the syndrome receded as kidney function rose back to normal and urine protein loss stopped. But this is very unusual. Most patients with chronic renal failure do not have the nephrotic syndrome, and few patients with the nephrotic syndrome and low glomerular filtration rate ever recover normal function.

Getting a Predialysis Program Funded

This book makes a case for a pre–end-stage renal disease program. The government has mounted an education program but has not seriously considered supporting predialysis care by payments to physicians (other than through existing Medicare and Medicaid programs). Keeping someone off dialysis should be rewarded at least as much as keeping someone on dialysis, but the government, having already incurred costs far exceeding earlier projections for the ESRD program, is not about to initiate yet another program. However, a recently enacted amendment to the Medicare legislation (Section 105, HR 5543) authorizes reimbursement for care by a nutritionist prior to the initiation of dialysis.

Perhaps someday the wisdom of government support for predialysis care by physicians will become apparent. This would not only reduce the cost of treatment of chronic kidney disease by both programs combined, but would also lead to an increased rate of rehabilitation of patients with kidney disease. The government also could play an important part in facilitating nondirected kidney donation for transplantation (see Chapter 20), reducing the number of patients on dialysis. These combined initiatives could, at least in theory, reduce the number of patients on dialysis to a handful.

In the next chapter, we'll scrutinize the kind of treatment you may be getting from your health care team and see whether you are receiving the best care possible.

5

Step 1: Assess Your Current Treatment Plan

As you saw in the last chapter, I am advising that people with kidney disease follow a very-low-protein diet with supplemental amino acids and also pay close attention to other problems caused by kidney failure. In this chapter we will assess your current treatment and decide whether you are getting the best possible care for your disease. This may be difficult to discuss with your doctor, so first let's look at how doctors and patients should work together.

How to Work with Your Doctor

When I was growing up, doctors behaved very differently from the way they do today. For one thing, they went out of their way to suppress information about alternative diagnoses, risks of treatment, and prognoses. They did this because they felt that part of their job was to shoulder the anxiety related to these sometimes horrible possibilities and conceal them from the patient and patient's family. When a fatal outcome was likely, telling the patient was taboo.

This approach wasn't all bad. "Trust me, I'm a doctor" sounded better then than it does now; patients didn't expect to be told everything about their condition.

What would your response be to a doctor who said no more than: "Trust me"? Those who are older may be more inclined to accept this statement, but most of us would press for more information. Rather than asking patients to trust me blindly, I answer questions as best I can. If I don't have an answer, I tell patients quite frankly, then do my best to find out. Common sense tells us that no one doctor has all of the answers, and a doctor may even have some embarrassing gaps in his or her knowledge. However, in my experience, acknowledging that I don't have immediate and definitive answers usually increases a patient's confidence in my abilities. Where there are gaps of information, I can look up the correct answers and respond later. With modern computerized databases and search programs, it is easy for me to get abstracts of the latest published information on just about any medical topic (or combination of topics) within minutes. Reviewing these abstracts and summarizing them for a patient is relatively straightforward, except when the information is contradictory. But if contradictory findings do turn up, that's what I tell my patient. If doctors had clear-cut answers to every question, then there would be no need for further medical research.

There still are wide differences among physicians in the extent to which they try to explain various aspects of each patient's illness. Some continue to believe that patients really don't need to know such details. Others think their patients won't understand them. This attitude has contributed to the demand for articles in general consumer magazines and on health Web sites and in books like this one designed to explain treatment of various diseases in terms that patients can understand.

Some physicians are still made uneasy by patients who read up on their disease and/or proposed treatments and come to the office with a lot of difficult questions, or worse yet, with specific demands, for example, for specific drugs they have seen advertised. Patients want to trust their doctors, and to leave the anxiety to the doctor. But patients need to know that all of the possibilities have been taken into consideration, that their doctor is completely informed, and most of all, that he or she is really concerned about their welfare. Explain your motives and concerns to your doctor. It is hoped that your doctor will be willing to assist you in furthering your knowledge once she realizes you're not second-guessing her.

One patient of mine carried the research of his disease to extremes. He was very keen on second and third opinions. He has seen most nephrologists in the area and some in neighboring areas, and still spends over $100,000 annually in doctor's bills. Typically, he will ask Dr. B and Dr. C to comment on the recommendations of Dr. A, and then he makes his own decision as to what to do and which doctor to entrust his care to.

This sort of "doctor shopping" is hard for physicians to tolerate. It is more than asking for a second opinion. Getting a second opinion (which is reimbursed by many insurers) doesn't imply that a second opinion that sounds better will lead to a change of doctors. No physician wants to spend time justifying his or her diagnosis, prognosis, or recommendations in the face of contrary opinions from another physician, knowing that the patient may switch doctors if he or she doesn't like the answers.

I do want you to be a well-informed patient and to take the knowledge that you learn in this book to your doctor. Take the Assessment of Care Quiz below, and find out whether you are receiving the best care possible for your kidney failure. An outline of the treatment options that might help your disease is presented after the quiz. If your doctor is unresponsive to these options, discuss with him or her why that may be. If you do not feel comfortable with the answers, consider changing doctors.

The Assessment of Care Quiz

Take the following test to assess the quality of care that you are receiving from your doctor to treat your kidney failure. You will need access to your latest lab values from a recent exam. If you do not have a copy of this report, call your doctor's office to ask for a copy.

The first two questions are intended to ascertain if you have kidney failure and are not scored. Questions 3 through 14 are scored as 0 to 10 points each and are intended to assess the quality of care you are receiving.

1. *Do you have kidney disease?* As noted in Chapter 4, the quickest way to find out (although it is not infallible) is to check your urine for protein. Buy paper test strips from the pharmacy and hold a strip in your urinary stream. If you have protein or glucose in your urine, the color will change (see package insert). If the color doesn't change, you probably do not have kidney disease (or diabetes) and do not need to take

this quiz. If you do have protein or glucose in your urine that was not previously recognized, you may need to consult your doctor. But note that the transient appearance of protein in the urine can also be caused by vigorous exercise, infection, fever, or very high blood sugar. You may want to check it again before you consult your doctor.

2. *Do you have kidney failure?* Look up your blood serum (or blood plasma) creatinine concentration on your lab report. If several lab results show that it is repeatedly 2 mg per dl or higher, you probably have chronic kidney failure and require medical care. Take the rest of this quiz to see if you are getting adequate care. If your creatinine concentration is lower than 2 mg per dl, you may not have kidney failure and do not need to take this quiz. If your creatinine concentration is higher than the upper level of normal (which varies somewhat in different laboratories, but is always printed on the lab report) but is less than 2 mg per dl, get it checked again after a month or so. If it remains in this range, consult your physician. Note that some people show elevated creatinine levels long before they show protein in their urine.

3. *Is your blood pressure well regulated?* It should be less than 130/80. If it is, give yourself 10 points. If only the first value (the systolic pressure) meets this target, score 5 points. If only the second value (the diastolic pressure) meets this target, score 5 points. (See Chapter 9.)

4. *Do you have any symptoms of kidney failure (such as fatigue, muscle cramps, itching, nausea, or vomiting)?* If so, you already may have been advised by a dietitian to eat a low-protein diet or a very-low-protein diet with a supplement of essential amino acids. If so (whether you have symptoms or not), give yourself 10 points. (See Chapter 7.)

5. *Do you have severe anemia?* This can be measured by several tests; the most widely used is the hematocrit (the percentage of your blood that red cells occupy). If your hematocrit is less than 30 percent and you have symptoms such as fatigue or shortness of breath on exertion, you have severe anemia and you should be getting injections of a hormone that stimulates your bone marrow to produce more red cells. Injections of Epogen or Procrit will bring your hematocrit above 30 percent. If your hematocrit is less than 30 percent and you are getting injections of this hormone, award yourself 5 points. If your hematocrit is over 30 percent, give yourself 10 points. (See Chapter 11.)

6. *Are you receiving one of the many drugs that inhibit the formation or action of a hormone called angiotensin?* These are collectively called either angiotensin-converting enzyme inhibitors (ACE inhibitors) or angiotensin receptor blockers (ARBs). Many drugs are available in each of these classes. You may need to ask your doctor about this. If you are receiving one of these drugs, award yourself 10 points. If you were receiving one of them, but it was discontinued for some reason, or if your kidney disease is so severe (creatinine level over 4 mg per dl) that the use of these drugs would be dangerous, award yourself 10 points.

7. *Is your serum potassium being checked, and is it less than 5.5 millequivalents per liter?* If so, add 10 points to your score. (See Chapter 12.)

8. *Is your serum carbon dioxide (bicarbonate) concentration being checked, and is it over 20 millimolar?* If so, add 10 points to your score. (See Chapter 10.)

9. *Is your serum calcium concentration between 8.6 and 10.6 mg per dl?* If so, add 10 points to your score. (See Chapter 13.)

10. *Is your serum phosphorus concentration less than 5 mg per dl?* If so, add 10 points to your score. (See Chapter 13.)

11. *Is your serum cholesterol concentration less than 200 mg per dl?* If so, add 10 points to your score. (See Chapter 15.)

12. *Are your ankles swollen?* If so, you should be taking a diuretic drug. If you are, or if your ankles are not swollen, add 10 points to your score. (See Chapter 8.)

13. *If you are diabetic, is your hemoglobin A1C concentration less than 7 percent?* (Hemoglobin A1C is a form of hemoglobin that has combined with glucose; a prolonged elevation of blood glucose level causes this combination to occur.) If so, add 10 points. If you have IgA nephropathy and are receiving fish oil, add another 10 points. (This form of kidney disease represents an immune response to a protein, IgA, which is a specific immunoglobulin. It has been well established that this disease responds to fish oil treatment.) If you have neither of these disorders, you still get 10 points.

14. *Is your serum albumin concentration greater than 3.5 g per dl?* If so, award yourself another 10 points.

Quiz Scoring

Now add up your total score.

If you scored less than 15 points: You care is being neglected. You may rapidly progress to dialysis. You may also sustain a serious or fatal complication even before your kidneys fail. You may need to change doctors, or at least discuss the situation with your doctor.

If you scored between 15 and 45 points: Your care could be a lot better. You will probably not do well and may go on dialysis before long unless your care improves.

If you scored between 45 and 70 points: Clearly you are receiving some attention, but some things could be improved that may affect your outcome.

If you scored greater than 70 points: Your physician is trying hard. Perhaps he or she could do even better. Care like this may stop progression of your kidney disease for years or even for the indefinite future.

If you scored 120 points: A perfect score. Congratulations to you and to your physician!

Treatment Options

Now we get to the good part: how we can best treat your kidney failure and make improvements in your quality of life for now and into the future. It can start as early as today. Here is a quick summary of the steps we are going to explore.

The following treatment options are considered in this book:

- *Eat a low-protein diet.* I strongly encourage you to explore going on a very-low-protein diet, supplemented with essential amino acids (or better yet, with ketoacids, although these are not currently available in the United States). We will discuss the results that you might expect from following such a diet. At the very least, your symptoms (if you have any) will decrease or disappear; at best, the progression of your kidney failure may stop, whether you have symptoms or not. (This statement is admittedly based for the most part on anecdotal evidence, but it is exemplified by the case reports in Chapter 22.)

- *Optimize your salt and water balance.* Regulating the intake of fluids and of salt and taking diuretics will help you to minimize signs of heart failure. This particular treatment isn't hard to do, but may require the involvement of your doctor.

- *Control your high blood pressure.* This critical step is often overlooked, yet we now know that controlling blood pressure may reduce protein loss in the urine, bringing levels into the normal range. It also may stop the decline of kidney function. In most patients, the right combination of drugs and good medical advice can normalize blood pressure. Again, your doctor needs to be involved.

- *Treat acidosis.* Acidosis is excessive acid in the body fluids, and is a common complication of kidney failure. Treatment is simple with over-the-counter medication (sodium bicarbonate) and may make you feel better. You may need to take more diuretic drugs to counteract the increased sodium load from the medication.

- *Treat anemia and iron deficiency.* Anemia, which is seen in about half of patients with renal failure, can cause shortness of breath on exertion or even outright heart failure, but is now quite easy to treat. Iron deficiency, which also is common, especially after treatment of anemia, may cause fatigue and other symptoms. It may also aggravate anemia, and may be a bit harder to treat.

- *Treat high serum potassium.* Ask your doctor when you should be concerned about serum potassium concentration and what you can do about it. High serum potassium is quite common, especially in patients on newer drugs for high blood pressure. It is very dangerous but readily treated, once recognized.

- *Supplement with calcium and restrict phosphorus intake.* Calcium supplementation (a universal need in patients with kidney failure) and phosphorus restriction measures are easy to put into effect and play a role in preventing bone disease. Adding vitamin D in its active form is very effective in raising serum calcium, but it is easy to overdo, and your kidneys will suffer as a consequence.

- *Watch out for gout.* Find out how to prevent gout from developing and what to do if it develops. Gout is a common and potentially distressing complication. Treating patients with kidney failure for gout is very different from treating gout in the absence of kidney failure.

- *Treat your high cholesterol.* Ask your doctor how and when to treat high serum cholesterol and/or triglyceride levels. Not only can these contribute to heart attacks (with or without kidney disease), but they also may play a role in the progression of kidney failure.

- *Measure the progression of your kidney failure* (the rate of decline in your kidney function). Measuring kidney function used to be a major undertaking, but now it can be accomplished very easily. See Chapter 17 for detailed information.

Each of the conditions just mentioned can cause major problems for patients with kidney failure, and all respond, to some degree, to treatment. We will be reviewing each one in the coming chapters so that you will have a full understanding of their importance. Other important issues that we will explore are:

- How to effectively slow the progression of kidney failure. Different measures are indicated in different kidney diseases.

- Dietary treatment of the nephrotic syndrome (large amounts of protein in the urine and a low level of protein in the serum). This syndrome, which is different from kidney failure, is commonly treated by high doses of steroids, but changes in diet alone bring about startling improvement in some patients and are much safer.

- Which drugs to avoid and which are safe. This list is one you should know and keep in mind, especially since many of these drugs are available without a doctor's prescription.

- Transplantation as a preferable alternative to dialysis, if you can arrange it.

- When to opt for dialysis. There may come a time, despite all of these measures, when the only answer is dialysis; the question is, how do you know when the time has come?

These issues are important. Although many internists are aware of the conditions just mentioned and how they can be treated, few initiate treatment, probably because they are encouraged to refer kidney patients to a nephrologist. The nephrologist, in turn, is likely to start you on dialysis as soon as possible, since a government-funded program pays for treatment, and early dialysis is widely believed to be the best and most appropriate treatment. Unfortunately, that is often not the case.

In the next chapter, we explore the lifestyle habits that affect your kidney failure.

6

Step 2: Make Lifestyle Changes

Let's take a look at your current lifestyle choices. Many choices may make you vulnerable to kidney disease and, if you already have it, will worsen the effects of kidney failure on your body and your symptoms. Yet there are some things that you can do to make yourself feel better. Here are the important things to consider as you lead your daily life.

Alcohol

Many laypeople believe alcohol is harmful to the kidneys. I am not sure how this notion arose, unless it is a result of confusing the liver with the kidneys. It is true that alcohol causes an increase in urine flow, but this does no harm to the kidneys, at least when moderate amounts of alcohol are ingested. It may cause some degree of dehydration— one component of a hangover.

As far as I know, there is no direct evidence for any adverse effect of moderate alcohol intake on the kidneys, other than indirectly through the occurrence of metabolic disorders such as potassium or magnesium deficiency or metabolic acidosis.

However, a recent epidemiological study, conducted by telephone, has shown that people who by their own accounts consume more than two drinks per day are more likely to have end-stage renal disease than people who drink less. The authors of the study controlled for differences in age, race, sex, income, use of opiates, cigarette smoking, history of diabetes, and consumption of moonshine (home-distilled whiskey). This association suggests, but does not prove, that heavy alcohol intake harms the kidneys. A lower intake of alcohol did not appear to be harmful. As the study's authors note, "Because these results are based on self-reports in a case-control study, they should be seen as preliminary." No studies have compared the relative dangers to the kidneys of beer, wine, and hard liquor.

Alcoholic drinks generally contain no protein and therefore could be viewed as a useful source of calories on a low-protein diet. If excess intake is not a problem, alcohol is a desirable component of a low-protein diet.

Smoking

Abundant evidence has been published establishing that smoking hastens the progression of kidney disease, especially in men. In patients with high blood pressure or with diabetes who do not yet show signs of renal disease, smoking increases the likelihood of abnormal urinary protein excretion, a precursor of renal failure. In a type of connective tissue disease called lupus, which commonly damages the kidneys, smokers progress to the end stage twice as fast as nonsmokers. When healthy nondiabetic individuals with normal blood pressure are screened by measurement of serum creatinine level and urinary protein, abnormally elevated levels of both are found more commonly in men (but not women) who are long-term smokers, according to a recent Australian study. These observations suggest that smoking may cause kidney damage.

As a patient with kidney disease, it is imperative that you take steps to cut smoking out of your life. In addition to nicotine patches and gum, many good programs can help. Call the American Lung Association for more information on quitting smoking, and find out about local programs in your community Local hospitals may offer similar programs.

Drugs

As mentioned in Chapter 5 and as discussed in greater detail in Chapter 19, analgesic abuse is a common cause of kidney failure, especially in Switzerland and Australia. Another cause is heroin, which, when injected intravenously, can lead to a severe and rapidly progressive form of renal failure. Whether this disorder is attributable to heroin itself or to a contaminant has not been established. Lithium, prescribed to treat bipolar disorder, also can induce renal failure.

Exercise

There is no reason for people with kidney failure to avoid strenuous activity. Patients can improve their exercise capacity considerably with regular workouts. Symptoms diminish and quality of life improves. When predialysis patients regularly exercised for four months, breathing capacity, muscular strength, and blood pressure all improved. There is no evidence, however, that exercise can defer dialysis; current evidence indicates that progression is unaffected. The general health benefits of regular exercise have been widely publicized and include lowering blood pressure, lowering blood cholesterol level, and weight loss.

In the next chapter, we move on to look at the cornerstone of predialysis kidney failure treatment, the low-protein diet.

7

Step 3: Follow a Low-Protein Diet

Before we discuss the low-protein diet that can be so beneficial in patients with kidney failure, let's look at why we need to eat the way we do.

We all need calories for energy. Our caloric requirements vary with our size, gender, and activity levels. It is possible to calculate your caloric requirement, based on these factors. But two much simpler approaches are to quit eating when you are no longer hungry, and to watch your weight.

Don't be fooled by the many things that can make you accumulate or lose fluid (and therefore weight) without flesh. One of these is salt, which we'll discuss fully in Chapter 8. People who have substantial accumulation of retained salt and water cannot use their weight as an index of their caloric needs. Ankle swelling is an early hallmark of this problem. Less common is water retention or deficit without accompanying salt or water deficit, which we'll also discuss in Chapter 8; this is usually a short-lived problem. Another is fluid accumulation caused by air travel, which takes a few days to recede. Obviously acute illnesses, especially diarrheal disease, can cause temporary weight loss owing to fluid loss.

Some people can eat all they want to and never gain or lose weight. They are very fortunate. No one knows what accounts for this. As far as I know, there is no measure of what fraction of the population they comprise, but we all know such people.

There are four possible food sources of energy: alcohol, protein, fat, and carbohydrate. Alcohol theoretically contains 7 calories per gram, but, for reasons only partially understood, in fact provides little energy. Fat contains 9 calories per gram; carbohydrate and protein each contain 4 calories per gram.

Alcohol

Alcohol, of course, is detrimental to anyone if ingested in excess; yet alcohol seems to help protect against coronary artery disease if it is ingested in relatively small amounts. Obviously people can get along fine without it too.

Protein

Everyone needs to consume a minimum quantity of the eight essential amino acids (the building blocks of protein). Our bodies cannot synthesize them. Twelve other amino acids used in protein synthesis, called nonessential amino acids, can be made in the body. They do not need to be consumed. Most proteins contain all 20 amino acids in differing proportions. We each need about 40 g of protein a day. Otherwise our bodies, which break down proteins continuously, cannot replenish them, and signs of protein deficiency will develop. Some dietary protein sources, such as eggs, contain these eight essential amino acids in nearly the optimal proportions for supporting protein synthesis, but other protein sources may not.

If these eight amino acids are ingested as such, in pure form, in appropriate dosage, no protein at all in the diet is needed for nutritional purposes. Pure amino acids have an unpleasant taste, but they do the job.

Fat

High intake of fat, as everyone knows, promotes all sorts of problems. A desirable goal is some 30 to 50 g per day of fat—far less than most Americans eat now. Chapter 15 discusses the various types of fats.

Carbohydrate

Carbohydrate is almost always the principle source of energy in our diets. The two main types, from the nutritional point of view, are simple sugars (like sucrose) and complex carbohydrates (like starch). Earlier the difference between these two types was thought to be especially important to diabetics, because simple sugars were thought to cause a more rapid rise in blood glucose levels than complex carbohydrates. This turns out to be incorrect; *all* carbohydrates raise blood glucose levels at the same rate. The other foods you eat in combination with the carbohydrate can make a big difference in sugar metabolism. Fats, in particular, slow down absorption. Both simple and complex carbohydrates yield the same energy, 4 calories per gram.

For most of us, protein provides about one-fifth of our total energy intake; fat a somewhat higher proportion; carbohydrate provides the rest.

So how should a person with kidney failure who wants to stay off dialysis consume these various sources of energy?

A simple dietary treatment used for about 100 years produces good results in patients with kidney failure—the low-protein diet pioneered by Franz Volhard, who wrote in 1918 that "in patients with chronic renal failure it is often possible to postpone the increase of serum urea concentration for a long time, reducing the nitrogen intake to 3 to 5 g. Sometimes we have succeeded in reducing considerably high serum urea concentrations. Consequently, the first uremic symptoms disappeared." (Volhard did not give amino acids, which we recommend here, because they were not available at that time.)

For reasons as yet unknown, high-protein foods aggravate several aspects of kidney failure, including the symptoms, and probably also the rate of decline of kidney function as the disease progresses. We don't know why this is true. The answer is not simply that high-protein foods generate more urea for the kidneys to dispose of. As noted in Chapter 3, the symptoms and signs of kidney failure are very poorly correlated with the degree of accumulation of urea in the blood, so that can't be it. Some of the hormones that contribute to kidney damage are stimulated by a high protein intake; that may be one reason why high-protein foods aggravate kidney failure, but it cannot be the entire explanation, because drugs are available that can block each of these hormones. Since the essential amino acids don't seem to cause these ill effects, it is conceivable that one or more of the nonessential amino acids of protein may do so. Other possibilities include substances besides amino acids found in high-protein foods, such as phosphorus-containing compounds, fatty materials, or various trace substances. Sorting out this puzzle may take some time.

A protein-restricted diet is the cornerstone of a predialysis treatment plan. High protein foods include meat, chicken, eggs, milk, and milk products, such as cheese. While it may be difficult to imagine life without enjoying these foods, perhaps it's better to concentrate on the fact that by reducing the amounts of protein in your diet, you may reduce markedly the uncomfortable symptoms of kidney failure, and the progression of your disease may slow as well. These two factors should encourage you to make the change. People with kidney failure also should avoid star fruit; there is evidence that this fruit can injure diseased or even normal kidneys.

As I've mentioned earlier in this book, most patients with chronic renal failure progress to the end stage without ever having received instruction on a low-protein diet. Some will report that their doctors have advised them to "cut down on red meat." But unless a dietitian becomes involved in their care, this sort of haphazard instruction usually results in little or no net change in protein intake, because another high-protein food, such as chicken or fish, is substituted for meat. Few physicians have the training or knowledge required to instruct patients on a low-protein diet.

Getting Started on the Very-Low-Protein Diet

The best way to get started on a very-low-protein diet is to meet with a dietitian. Dietitians have a R.D. degree, meaning registered dietitian. People with this degree have met certain educational requirements in the field of nutrition. The American Dietetic Association is a good source for finding a dietitian in your area, if your doctor cannot recommend one. The dietitian will explore your eating habits and favorite foods, and will design for you a diet that meets your requirements for calories and your limits for protein and phosphorus. He or she also will advise you on how to get supplemental essential amino acids (either as powder or as tablets), calcium carbonate, ferrous sulfate, zinc sulfate (or zinc gluconate), and multivitamins. (See Appendix 1.) You will be given some low-protein recipes that appeal to you. If, at the next visit, you are losing weight (and don't want to), you will be advised on how to increase your caloric intake. Third and subsequent visits will be provided only if you request them, or if there is evidence that you're having trouble getting or staying on the program.

The most important features of the very-low-protein diet are:

1. Severe restriction of protein intake (to about 21 g per day, in contrast with a usual intake of about 100 g per day). (See Table 1.)

2. Avoidance of high-phosphorus foods. (See Table 2 later in this chapter.)

3. Addition of an essential amino acid supplement as either tablets or powder, taken with meals (about 10 g per day). You must supplement your restricted protein intake with essential amino acids. Eating this diet without taking a supplement of essential amino acids is bound to cause protein deficiency in time.

The dietitian will prescribe how many calories you need. Many patients feel they're not getting enough to eat at first and feel hungry. A second conference with the dietitian usually corrects the problem. A few patients, however, tend to lose weight. Others tend to gain, because they never feel entirely satisfied and regularly consume more than recommended. Usually, but not invariably, these problems can be corrected by further consultation with the dietitian.

Those who want to lose weight can do so on this diet by gradually reducing their caloric intake. It is important to take it slow, because drastically reducing your caloric intake can lead to the loss of lean tissue. When you reduce your caloric intake gradually, your body burns fat stores for energy, and does not consume much lean tissue. However, when you cut back drastically, lean tissue eventually is burned in substantial amounts. Not only does this reduce body protein stores, but it also tends to defeat the goal of protein restriction. Total fasting, for example, exhausts body fat stores at first, with only modest depletion of protein stores, resulting in a fall in urea formation. But eventually fat stores become depleted and urea formation (derived from burning protein stores) rises back to normal or above normal.

The most difficult aspect of this diet is eating out. If there is no low-protein option on the menu, ask the server to omit the meat (or fish or poultry) entrée and to bring everything else. Another option is to utilize the salad bar liberally, avoiding only items like beans, cheese, and bacon bits.

People with diabetes will find that this diet does not compromise any of their goals for controlling blood glucose levels. They can replace the protein calories deleted from the diet with complex carbohydrates such as pastas or starch.

People with high cholesterol may be alarmed at this diet's fat content. Surprisingly, patients' serum cholesterol usually falls on this diet, despite its relatively high fat content.

Let's get specific about the kind of foods you should be eating in a low-protein diet. Table 1 lists common foods (and special low-protein products) in order of their ratio of protein to calories. You're encouraged to eat foods in Category I, which have a low protein content. You should avoid the foods in Category III. They are included for informational purposes. Category II foods are intermediate, and can be consumed in limited amounts. Sticking to the foods in Category I or Category II will optimize caloric intake, thus filling you up more quickly, while minimizing protein intake. As you will note, many appealing foods are in Category I and are okay to consume.

TABLE 1. PROTEIN CONTENT IN RELATION TO CALORIES

Category I: Foods with less than 0.6 g protein per 100 cal

Fats and oils

Fruit juices

Sugar, honey, jelly

Low-protein products available from specialized sources:
Products Distributed by Cambrooke Foods
(www.cambrookefoods.com; 508-601-1640)
    Artisan Bread

Bagel
Energy Bars
Low Protein Cheddar Cheese
Low Protein Jalapeno Singles
Low Protein Mozzarella Shreds
Munchy Bites
Whitehall LP American Single
Whitehall LP Swiss Cheese

Products Distributed by Dietary Specialties
(www.dietspec.com; 888-MENU-123)

Bread and crackers
Cookies
Imitation Macaroni and Cheeses
Imitation Rice
LP Gelled Dessert Mix
LP Plantain Chips
Pasta
Peanut Butter Flavored Spread
Porridge
Sauce Mixes
Vance's Dairifree Beverage Mix
Wel-Plan Baking Mixes
Wise Onion Rings

Products Distributed by Ener-G-Foods
(www.ener-g.com; 800-331-5222)

Doughnuts
Egg Replacer
LP Pizza Crust
Potato Mix

Products Distributed by Med Diet Labs
(www.med-diet.com; 800-633-5550)

Broth, Soups, Gravies
Coating Mixes
Dessert
Pizza with Cheese Topping

Products Distributed by Scientific Hospital Supplies
(www.shsna.com; 888-LOPROGO)

Breakfast Cereal Loops
Broth, Soups, Sauces, Gravies
Crackers
Drink Mix
Loprofin Baking Mix
Pasta
Sweet Biscuits
Wafers

Category II: Foods Containing Significant but Acceptable Amounts of Protein
(Consume those near the beginning of this list freely, but those near the end sparingly.)

FOOD	*g protein per 100 cal*
Apple	0.3
Rhubarb	0.4
Butter	0.5
Pineapple	0.6
Dates	0.7
Apricots	0.7
Grapes	0.9
Tapioca	0.9
Potato chips	0.9
Blueberries	1.0
Grapefruit	1.0
Hash brown potatoes (cooked in oil)	1.0
Pear	1.0
Peach	1.2
Banana	1.2
Figs	1.2
Avocado	1.2
Frosted flakes	1.3
Coconut	1.3
Pecans	1.4
Sweet potato	1.5
Corn flakes	1.5
Strawberries	1.5
French fried potatoes	1.6
Doughnut	1.6

FOOD	g protein per 100 cal
Watermelon	1.6
Cherries	1.7
Orange	1.8
Filberts	1.9
Rice	1.9
Rice Krispies	1.9
Blackberries	1.9
Cream cheese	2.1
Honeydew	2.1
Flour	2.2
Brazil nuts	2.2
Cream (half and half)	2.3
Walnuts	2.3
Ice cream	2.3
Carrots	2.6
Squash	2.6
Potato	2.7
Noodles	2.7
Wheaties	2.7
Waffle	2.8
Corn	3.0
Cashews	3.1
Almonds	3.1
Turnips	3.2
Pistachios	3.2
Cream of wheat	3.2
White bread	3.2
Whole wheat bread	3.4
Bran flakes	3.4
Beets	3.4
Onions	3.6
Cheerios	3.6
English muffin	3.6
Macaroni	3.7
Spaghetti	3.9
Sausage	3.9
Lettuce	4.0
Tomato	4.0

continued

FOOD	g protein per 100 cal
Frankfurter	4.1
Peanut butter	4.2
Sunflower seeds	4.3
Peanuts	4.4
Peppers	4.5
Eggplant	4.5
Bacon	4.9

Category III: Foods to be Avoided (High-Protein Foods)

FOOD	g protein per 100 cal
Celery	5.0
Cabbage	5.0
Artichokes	5.4
Whole milk	5.4
Beans, green	5.5
Lima beans	6.1
American cheese	6.3
Cheddar cheese	6.4
Cream cheese	7.1
Lentils	7.2
Peas	7.3
Swiss cheese	7.5
Brussels sprouts	7.8
Egg	8.1
Yogurt	8.3
Cauliflower	8.3
Broccoli	8.7
Asparagus	8.7
Spinach	8.8
Skim milk	10.0
Mushrooms	10.0
Buttermilk	10.0
Veal	11.7
Pork	11.9
Sardines	12.1
Oysters	13.3
Lamb	13.6
Beef	14.5

FOOD	*g protein per 100 cal*
Cottage cheese	15.0
Chicken	15.4
Fish	17.0
Turkey	17.3
Lobster	17.9
Scallops	21.7

Getting Low-Protein Foods at the Store or by Catalog

Many specially prepared low-protein foods are available in stores and by mail. They make counting protein consumption easier, although whether you'll like the taste enough to eat them regularly is anyone's guess. Certainly they add significantly to the cost of the diet. Low-protein bread is the most generally useful low-protein food, preferably made at home in an automatic bread maker. Toasting improves its flavor. In my experience, this bread may make the difference between a person's success or failure on a low-protein diet. Bread is a staple in most people's diets, but regular bread contains too much protein (about 2 g per slice). Low-protein bread contains only 0.2 g per slice, so you can eat many slices without exceeding the protein limit

Here is a recipe for low-protein bread made in a breadmaking machine, reproduced by permission of Scientific Hospital Supplies. This recipe makes a 2-pound loaf.

Low-Protein Bread

1¾ cup water (lukewarm)
2 tbsp vegetable oil
500 g (1 box) Loprofin Baking Mix®
1½ tsp powdered Coffee Mate®
1 tbsp sugar
½ tsp salt
1 packet (7 g) yeast (included in the Loprofin Baking Mix®)

Add ingredients according to the instructions for your bread machine. Use the "white bread, dry milk" setting. Bake approximately 4 hours. Yield: 12 servings (1 serving = 1 slice)

Nutrition information:

Calories	2,013 per recipe; 168 per serving
Protein:	4.67 per recipe; 0.39 g per serving

Eating these foods will optimize caloric intake while minimizing protein intake. But knowing which foods to consume is only part of the process. If you don't know how to prepare these foods in ways that appeal to you, you'll never eat them. A former patient of mine, Tim Ahlstrom, collected some low-protein recipes in his book entitled *The Kidney Patient's Book*, which is now out of print. Two of the recipes are repeated here.

Murray West's Baked Peppers, Onions, and Potatoes

    5 red or green peppers cored, seeded, and chopped into 1-inch dice
    5 potatoes, peeled and quartered
    1 medium onion, quartered
    1 cup olive oil
    pepper to taste

Preheat oven to 425 degrees.

Mix together all ingredients in a baking dish, taking care that all the vegetables are covered with the olive oil. Lots of any kind of pepper— black, red, dried chili, fresh chili—adds zest.

Bake for about 20 to 25 minutes. Yield: 4 servings

Nutrition Information:
    Protein: 4 g
    Calories: 660
    Phosphorus: 99 mg

Sandra Watt's Braised Broccoli

    ⅔ cup broccoli, fresh or frozen
    1 tbsp peanut oil (or other vegetable oil)
    2 slices fresh ginger root, thinly sliced
    1 tbsp oyster sauce
    ½ tbsp Soy sauce
    1 tsp sugar
    ½ tsp sesame oil
    ½ cup liquid from blanching the broccoli
    1 tsp cornstarch

Cut the broccoli into bite-size pieces. Bring lightly salted water to a boil in a saucepan. Add the broccoli and blanch it for 1 minute. Drain in a colander, but save ½ cup of the liquid.

Heat the peanut oil in a wok and stir-fry the broccoli and ginger root for 1 minute. Add oyster sauce, soy sauce, sugar, sesame oil, and cooking liquid. Bring to a boil.

Mix the cornstarch with 1 tbsp cold water and stir into the liquid until it thickens slightly. Add broccoli, toss, and serve. Yield: 1 serving
Nutrition information:

Protein: 5 g
Calories: 333
Phosphorus: 123 mg

More low-protein recipes have been developed for people suffering from a totally different disease: phenylketonuria. In this relatively common congenital disorder, patients cannot metabolize phenylalanine (an essential amino acid) owing to an enzyme defect, and it accumulates in body fluids. Mental retardation can result. All proteins contain phenylalanine. Therefore, the mainstay of treatment is a low-protein diet, supplemented by an amino acid mixture lacking phenylalanine. Initially this regimen was recommended only for infants and children, but gradually it has become recommended "for life." Virginia E. Schuett has written a book containing hundreds of low-protein recipes for such patients. I recommend it highly.

High Phosphate Foods—Warning

As we explained in greater detail in Chapter 13, phosphorus (as inorganic phosphate) may accumulate in the blood of people with kidney failure, and can exacerbate kidney damage. Most patients following the very-low-protein diet do not have high blood phosphate levels, because low-protein foods are typically low-phosphorus foods as well. But occasionally people have a problem with high serum phosphate despite following the very-low-protein diet. They should consume high-phosphorus foods (see later) in limited amounts or avoid them entirely. Common foods in order of their phosphorus-to-calorie ratios are listed in Table 2. The reason for listing them in this order is the same as the reason for listing protein content in relation to calories: You are liable to limit your intake of these foods by satiety.

Most of this food phosphorus is in chemical forms other than inorganic phosphate, but it becomes a source of inorganic phosphate when eaten. This list of foods resembles the list in Table 1. However, there are important differences, because not all of the phosphorus in common foods is linked with proteins.

The only people who need to concern themselves with this second list are those whose serum phosphate concentration remains above normal (greater than 5 mg per dl) despite limiting their protein intake to 0.3 g per kg per day. These people should avoid, or consume only rarely and in small quantities, foods at the end of Table 2. Also, a number of instant beverages, sold as powders, contain added calcium phosphate to make the powder free-flowing; also avoid these (check the labels). Taking these measures will almost always bring serum phosphate concentration down into the normal range after a few weeks.

TABLE 2. PHOSPHORUS CONTENT OF COMMON FOODS ARRANGED IN ORDER (APPROXIMATELY) OF MG PHOSPHORUS PER 100 CALORIES

Food	Portion	Mg Phosphorus per Portion
Category I: Low-Phosphorus Foods		
Vegetable oils	1 tbsp	0
Margarine	1 tbsp	2
Whipping cream	1 tbsp	9
Mayonnaise	1 tbsp	4
White wine	1 glass	13
Corn flakes	1 cup	8
Avocado	½ cup	32
Apple	1	11
Pineapple	½ cup	6
Apricot	1	8
Coconut, shredded	1 cup	9
Orange	½ cup	18
Lemon meringue pie	1 sector	7
Red wine	1 glass	13
Pear	1	18
Dates	½ cup	56
Chocolate	1 oz.	50
Watermelon	½ cup	8
Grapes	1 cup	12

Food	Portion	Mg Phosphorus per Portion
Potato chips	10 chips	25
Rice	1 cup	56
Flour	2 tbsp	15
Butter	1 tsp	1
Grapefruit juice	1 cup	38
Banana	1	10
Boiled potato	1	41
Coca-Cola	12 oz	60
Pancakes	1 4-in cake	70
Macaroni	1 cup	70
Mustard	1 tsp	4
Rice Krispies	1 cup	39
Plum	1	5
Ketchup	3 tbsp	16
Figs	1	11
Honeydew melon	½ cup	14
Baked potato	1 small	51
Frankfurter	1	60
Beer	12 oz	50
Special K	1 cup	28
Tangerine	1	15
Peach	1	19
Sweet potato	½ cup	60
Prune	1	5
Sirloin steak	1 oz	68
Duck	1 oz	67
Ice cream	1 cup	150
Peanuts	2 tbsp	122
American cheese	1 oz	219
Bacon	1 slice	17
Sausage	1 oz	44
Tuna	1 oz	66
Orange	1 cup	36
Pork	1 oz	87
Grapefruit	1 cup	32
Lamb	1 oz	62
Chicken	1 oz	79

continued

Food	Portion	Mg Phosphorus per Portion
Mushrooms	1 cup	81
Blackberries	1 cup	28
Whole wheat bread	1 slice	57
White bread	1 slice	24
Strawberries	1 cup	32
Carrots, cooked	1 cup	48
Corn	1 cob	69

Category II: Moderate-Phosphorus Foods

Food	Portion	Mg Phosphorus per Portion
Raisins	1 cup	168
Oatmeal	1 cup	136
Peanut butter	2 tbsp	200
Cod	1 oz	78
Shredded Wheat	1 cup	158
Puffed Wheat	1 cup	48
Raspberries	1 cup	28
Turkey	1 oz	67
Onions, cooked	1 cup	62
Cantaloupe	1 cup	26
Cheddar cheese	1 oz	136
Green beans	1 cup	46
Haddock	1 oz	70
Milk	1 cup	228
Tomato, 2-in. diameter	1	25
Egg, large	1	103
Cottage cheese, creamed	1 cup	152
Salmon, fresh cooked	1 oz	117
Cabbage, fresh	1 cup	26
Peas	1 cup	158
Green pepper, fresh	1 cup	22
Brussels sprouts	1 cup	112
Radishes	1 cup	36
Calves' liver	1 oz	133
Lettuce	1 cup	118
Shrimp, cooked	1 oz	54
Lobster, cooked	1 oz	54
Cucumber	1 cup	26

Food	Portion	Mg Phosphorus per Portion
Sardines	1 oz	141
Artichokes	1	69
Coffee	6 oz	4
Tea	8 oz	10

Category III: High-Phosphorus Foods

Yogurt	1 cup	326
Skim milk	1 cup	234
Spinach, cooked	1 cup	68
Scallops	1 oz	95
Broccoli	1 cup	96
Rhubarb, cooked	1 cup	42
Cauliflower, cooked	1 cup	54
Okra	1 cup	66
Asparagus, fresh	1 cup	90
Oysters, raw	1 oz	91
Bran flakes	1 cup	125

Menu Plans

My dietitian, Nga Hong Brereton, with the assistance of another dietitian, Keena Andrews, has devised six days' worth of complete menu plans for the very-low-protein diet, which you can modify to suit your tastes.

Each menu consists of approximately 20 g protein and 2,200 calories. This is an average caloric requirement for a 70 kg (154 lb) male whose physical activity is also average—for example, a student who walks back and forth to classes. Most of these calories are used for basal metabolism (about 1,400); physical activity uses another 500, and the remainder is used in assimilating food. But many factors modify energy requirements: age, sex, body size and composition, genetic factors, energy intake, growth, pregnancy and lactation, coexisting pathological conditions, and ambient temperature. For a full presentation of caloric requirements, see *Recommended Dietary Allowances*, published by the National Academy Press. Note that supplemental amino acids are part of each meal.

MENU 1

Foods/Beverages	Calories	Protein (g)	Sodium (mg)	Phosphorus (mg)	Supplements
Breakfast					
¼ teaspoon salt with dried herbs to put in a salt shaker to use for all-day seasoning	0	0	589	0	5 Aminess or Aminess N tablets (690 mg each)
1 slice low-protein bread, toasted	110	0.3	280	24	
2 tablespoons margarine, unsalted	196	0.25	0	6	*or* 1 packet (3.5 g) Nutramine
1 tablespoon jam, regular or diabetic	48	0.14	8	2	*or*
½ medium banana	54	0.61	1	12	Nutramine T powder
½ cup cranberry with white grape juice	72	0.65	3	13	
Morning Snack					
½ cup Rice Dream®	60	0.5	45	N/A	1 Caltrate 600 tablet 1 Nephrocap
Lunch					
Sandwich:					5 Aminess or Aminess N tablets (690 mg each)
1 Cambrooke Low Protein Bagel®	304	0.2	760	N/A	
¼ avocado	70	0.86	4	18	
1 slice low-protein American cheese	60	0.7	230	N/A	*or*
2 leaves iceberg lettuce	2	0.16	1	3	1 packet (3.5 g) Nutramine
1 oz potato chips, unsalted	156	1.51	1	45	*or*
1 medium peach	42	0.69	0	12	Nutramine T powder
½ cup apple juice	68	0.12	4	9	
Dinner					
3 oz mushrooms, cooked	31	1.27	1	51	5 Aminess or Aminess N tablets
⅔ cup cooked white rice	487	10.07	4	161	

Foods/Beverages	Calories	Protein (g)	Sodium (mg)	Phosphorus (mg)	Supplements
½ cup green beans, fresh	18	0.93	6	19	(690 mg each) *or*
½ cup honey-glazed carrots	117	0.86	49	23	1 packet (3.5 g)
1 slice low-protein bread	110	0.3	280	N/A	Nutramine or Nutramine T powder
1 baked Granny Smith apple, including 5 raisins, 1 tablespoon brown sugar, and ½ cup ginger ale	198	0.27	20	16	1 Caltrate 600 tablet
1 cup chamomile tea	2	0	2	0	
Bedtime Snack					
1 bar (0.78 oz) Rice Krispies Treat®	86	0.43	81	8	
Total	2,291	20.82	2,368	>422	

MENU 2

Foods/Beverages	Calories	Protein (g)	Sodium (mg)	Phosphorus (mg)	Supplements
Breakfast					
1 4-inch-diameter regular frozen pancake	82	1.87	183	134	5 Aminess or Aminess N tablets (690 mg each) *or*
1 tablespoon low-salt Smart Beat Low Fat margarine®	22	0	1	0	1 packet (3.5 g)
1 tablespoon diet pancake syrup	17	0	67	4	Nutramine or
1 cup fresh strawberries	43	0.88	1	27	Nutramine T powder
1 cup weak tea, with lemon and Equal®	2	0	7	2	

MENU 2 *(CONTINUED)*

Foods/Beverages	Calories	Protein (g)	Sodium (mg)	Phosphorus (mg)	Supplements
Morning Snack					
1 packet Loprofin crackers®	140	0.1	N/A	N/A	1 Caltrate 600 tablet 1 Nephrocap
Lunch					
Low-protein rice mix:					5 Aminess
⅓ cup raw regular long-grain white rice	243	5.04	2	80	or Aminess N tablets (690 mg
⅓ cup low-protein rice, cooked per directions	210	0.2	17	N/A	each) *or*
2 tablespoons vegetable oil	241	0	0	0	1 packet (3.5 g)
2 tablespoons tomato paste	13	0.6	129	13	Nutramine or
1 cup vegetable broth	12	0.15	263	5	Nutramine
10 snow peas	14	1.07	1	18	T powder
1 fresh persimmon	118	0.97	2	29	
1 cup hot water with fresh ginger slices and Equal®	2	0	2	0	
Afternoon Snack					
½ cup watermelon	49	0.94	3	14	
Dinner					
2 cups cooked Chinese fried noodles mix:					5 Aminess or Aminess N tablets
2 bundles of clear noodles	349	2.91	61	64	*or* 1 packet
½ cup julienned carrot	28	0.66	22	28	(3.5 g)
1 cup shredded cabbage	13	0.76	9	12	Nutramine or
2 green onions	5	0	0	0	Nutramine
¼ cup safflower oil	477	0	0	0	T powder
3 tablespoons light soy sauce	25	2.47	1,594	53	1 Caltrate
Black pepper	0	0	0	0	600 tablet
1 orange	62	1.23	0	18	

Foods/Beverages	Calories	Protein (g)	Sodium (mg)	Phosphorus (mg)	Supplements
Bedtime Snack					
1 pear	98	0.65	0	18	
1 cup jasmine tea	2	0	7	2	
Total	2,262	20.5	2,373	521	

MENU 3

Foods/Beverages	Calories	Protein (g)	Sodium (mg)	Phosphorus (mg)	Supplements
Breakfast					5 Aminess or
1 cup Rice Krispies Cereal®	100	1.66	283	35	Aminess N
1 cup Coffee Rich®	410	0	148	1	tablets (690 mg each)
1 cup blueberries, fresh	81	0.97	9	15	*or*
½ cup apple juice	58	0.07	4	9	1 packet
1 cup coffee with	5	0.28	2	7	(3.5 g)
2 tablespoons Coffee Rich®	34	0	6	0	Nutramine or
2 teaspoons sugar	32	0	0	0	Nutramine T powder
Lunch					5 Aminess or
1 cup potato salad without egg	341	2.69	628	68	Aminess N tablets (690
1 medium croissant roll	259	4.59	76	65	mg each) *or*
2 teaspoons margarine, unsalted	65	0.08	0	2	1 packet
1 cup cantaloupe	56	1.41	14	27	(3.5 g)
12 oz clear soda (seltzer or 7-Up®)	147	0	41	0	Nutramine or Nutramine T powder
Dinner					5 Aminess or
Sandwich:					Aminess N
2 slices low-protein bread	220	0.6	560	N/A	tablets

MENU 3 *(CONTINUED)*

Foods/Beverages	Calories	Protein (g)	Sodium (mg)	Phosphorus (mg)	Supplements
2 medium slices tomato	8	0.34	4	10	(690 mg each) *or*
¼ avocado, sliced	70	0.86	4	18	1 packet
2 slices low-sodium bacon	73	3.86	130	43	(3.5 g) Nutramine
1 tablespoon mayonnaise	47	0.08	95	3	or Nutramine
Vegetable Soup:					T powder
1 cube low-sodium bouillon	18	0.96	3	6	
¼ cup low-protein macaroni, dry	67	0.1	N/A	10	
¼ cup frozen mixed vegetables	6	0.55	6	13	
Black pepper	0	0	0	0	
½ cup cranberry with white grape juice	72	0.65	3	N/A	
Bedtime Snack					
4 Loprofin Vanilla Cream Filled Wafers®	160	Trace	N/A	N/A	1 Caltrate 600 tablet 1 Nephrocap
Total	2,359	19.75	2,016	332	

MENU 4

Foods/Beverages	Calories	Protein (g)	Sodium (mg)	Phosphorus (mg)	Supplements
Breakfast					
1 medium Danish pastry (4¼-inch diameter)	511	4.81	157	65	5 Aminess or Aminess N tablets (690 mg each)
½ cup applesauce	97	0.23	4	9	
1 cup coffee with	5	0.28	2	7	*or*
¼ cup Coffee Rich®	67	0	13	0	1 packet (3.5 g) Nutramine or Nutramine T powder

Foods/Beverages	Calories	Protein (g)	Sodium (mg)	Phosphorus (mg)	Supplements
Morning Snack					
1 large peach	68	1.1	0	19	1 Caltrate 600 tablet 1 Nephrocap
Lunch					
Sandwich:					
2 slices low-protein bread	220	0.6	560	N/A	5 Aminess or Aminess N tablets (690
2 tablespoons mayonnaise	95	0.16	190	5	mg each) *or*
1 Amy Veggie Burger®	100	4.0	290	N/A	1 packet (3.5 g)
5 slices cucumber	4	0.20	1	7	Nutramine
2 slices onion	7	0.21	1	6	or
1 plum	36	0.52	0	7	Nutramine
½ cup Hawaiian Punch®	58	0	27	1	T powder
Dinner					
6 fluid oz white wine	124	0.35	0	25	5 Aminess or Aminess N
2 cups cooked low-protein pasta (from ⅕ packet)	360	0.6	17	N/A	tablets (690 mg each)
1 tablespoon olive oil	119	0	0	0	*or* 1 packet
¾ cup no-meat spaghetti sauce, low salt	144	2.94	65	64	(3.5 g) Nutramine or
Salad:					Nutramine
½ cup raw broccoli florets	12	1.31	12	29	T powder
½ medium cucumber, cubed	14	0.75	2	22	
¼ red bell pepper, sliced	8	0.26	1	6	
2 tablespoons chopped Vidalia onion,	8	0.23	12	28	
½ cup mayonnaise	589	0.72	0	5	
¼ cup white vinegar	8	0	2	0	
1 tablespoon sugar	48	0	1	0	

MENU 4 (CONTINUED)

Foods/Beverages	Calories	Protein (g)	Sodium (mg)	Phosphorus (mg)	Supplements
Low-protein garlic bread: ½ Cambrooke Artisan Bread Roll®, sliced	178	0.3	732	N/A	
¼ teaspoon unsalted butter powder (not garlic salt!)	102	0.12	0	3	
1 Granny Smith apple	70	0.4	0	3	
1 cup coffee substitute with ¼ cup Coffee Rich®	67	0	380	3	
1 teaspoon sugar	20	0	13	0	
Total	3,139	20.09	2,306	336	

MENU 5

Foods/Beverages	Calories	Protein (g)	Sodium (mg)	Phosphorus (mg)	Supplements
Breakfast					
½ cup canned peaches	54	0.55	5	13	5 Aminess or Aminess N tablets (690 mg each)
1 cup apple juice	136	0	7	17	
1 slice low-protein bread	110	0.3	280	N/A	*or*
1 teaspoon unsalted butter	34	0.04	1	1	1 packet (3.5 g)
1 tablespoon jam	48	0.14	8	2	Nutramine or Nutramine T powder
Lunch					
2 cups Cambrooke Macaroni and Cheese®	490	0.38	1104	N/A	5 Aminess or Aminess N tablets (690

Foods/Beverages	Calories	Protein (g)	Sodium (mg)	Phosphorus (mg)	Supplements
Salad:					mg each)
5 asparagus spears	15	1.62	2	30	or
5 slices cucumber	4	0.20	1	7	1 packet
5 cherry tomatoes	18	0.72	8	20	(3.5 g)
1 tablespoon Caesar					Nutramine
salad dressing	52	0.49	142	9	or
¾ cup apple pie	615	4.92	24	118	Nutramine
1 cup Hawaiian					T powder
Punch®	116	0	54	2	1 Caltrate
					600 tablet
					1 Nephrocap
Dinner					
1 serving vegetable					5 Aminess or
chili (see p. 192)	150	6.55	980	167	Aminess N
1 slice low-protein					tablets (690
bread	110	0.3	280	N/A	mg each)
1 pear	98	0.65	0	18	or
1 slice low-protein					1 packet
birthday cake					(3.5 g)
(see p. 193)	292	2.6	366	140	Nutramine
1 cup regular coffee	5	0.24	5	2	or
with: ¼ cup Coffee					Nutramine
Rich®	103	0	37	0	T powder
Total	2,450	19.7	3,304	>546	

MENU 6

Foods/Beverages	Calories	Protein (g)	Sodium (mg)	Phosphorus (mg)	Supplements
Breakfast					
1 cup corn flakes	102	1.84	298	11	5 Aminess or
½ cup Coffee Mate®	205	0	74	1	Aminess N
					tablets (690
					mg each)
					or
					1 packet (3.5 g)
					Nutramine
					or Nutramine
					T powder

MENU 6 (CONTINUED)

Foods/Beverages	Calories	Protein (g)	Sodium (mg)	Phosphorus (mg)	Supplements
Lunch					5 Aminess or
Peanut butter					Aminess N
sandwich:					tablets (690
2 slices low-protein					mg each)
bread	220	0.6	560	N/A	*or*
1 teaspoon peanut					1 packet
butter, unsalted	32	1.36	1	20	(3.5 g)
2 tablespoons grape					Nutramine
jelly	91	0.26	15	4	or
1 cup decaffeinated					Nutramine
coffee	5	0.24	5	2	T powder
					1 Caltrate
					600 tablet
					1 Nephrocap
Dinner					5 Aminess or
6 oz white wine	124	0.35	14	25	Aminess N
2 slices low-protein					tablets (690
bread, toasted	220	0.6	560	N/A	mg each)
1 oz eggplant	21	0.3	40	7	*or*
1 thin slice roast					1 packet
turkey (35 g)	49	10.6	19	75	(3.5 g)
½ cup cranberry and					Nutramine
pineapple relish					or
(see p. 195)	55	0.2	4	4	Nutramine
½ cup green beans					T powder
with 1 teaspoon					
olive oil	16	0.8	70	17	
1 cup low-protein					
pasta salad:					
1 cup cooked					
Loprofin® pasta	420	0.3	34	N/A	
1 black olive, thinly					
sliced	5	0.05	35	0	
5 cherry tomatoes	18	0.72	8	20	
1 scallion, thinly					
sliced	18	0.09	1	2	
2 fresh basil leaves,					
finely chopped	62	0.34	133	13	

Foods/Beverages	Calories	Protein (g)	Sodium (mg)	Phosphorus (mg)	Supplements
1 tablespoon Italian salad dressing	120	0	0	0	
1 tablespoon safflower oil	430	0.9	20	35	
Black pepper	0	0	0	0	
1 slice low-protein pumpkin pie (see p. 194)	20	0.18	1	0	
2 tablespoons Cool Whip®	5	0.24	5	2	
1 cup coffee with: 2 tablespoons coffee creamer	51	0	18	0	
1 teaspoon sugar	16	0	0	0	
Total	2,254	19.9	1,910	>230	

Diet for Patients with Kidney Stones

People with kidney stones need to follow one of several totally different diets, depending on the kind of stones they have. They may be advised to avoid high calcium-foods, high oxalate foods (such as spinach, rhubarb, and beets), or high-purine foods (liver and kidney); usually they also are advised to restrict dietary protein, though not as severely as people with kidney failure.

Motivation for the Very-Low-Protein Diet

This diet is very likely a radical departure from the diet you're accustomed to. Many favorite foods may become taboo. Furthermore, some patients never feel satisfied on this diet and are chronically hungry. It certainly takes some getting used to, particularly when you must keep track of every gram of protein that you eat. The best advice I have to offer is to experiment with it; keep track of recipes and meal planning so that ultimately you're eating meals that appeal to you. Patients often aren't sufficiently motivated to go on this diet until they experience the symptoms of kidney failure. Nevertheless, the diet may be beneficial before symptoms develop, especially for people who lose a lot of protein in their urine; dietary protein restriction reduces urinary protein excretion. (See Chapter 18.) It may also be beneficial in children with chronic renal failure.

Some patients won't consider following such a diet. Other patients are determined to try a supplemented very-low-protein diet even before they become symptomatic, in the hope that the progression of their kidney failure may slow. There is certainly no evidence that protein restriction accelerates the progression of kidney failure, and there is no reason to fear any adverse consequences, such as protein deficiency, provided that the diet is properly supplemented with essential amino acids and is prescribed by a dietitian.

The Low-Protein Diet
Versus Other Diets

Carmelo Giordano and Sergio Giovannetti in Italy first reported on the use of very-low-protein diets supplemented by essential amino acids in chronic renal failure 40 years ago. Although their clinical results were impressive, their diets, which contained very small amounts of protein, were almost intolerable. Jonas Bergström and his associates in Sweden were the first to recommend what I am now referring to as the very-low-protein diet. This diet contains about 22 g per day of protein for an average-size individual, much less than the average U.S. intake of about 100 g per day of protein. The reason this very low intake of protein is acceptable to most patients is that the sources of dietary protein are not restricted; any food that stays within these limits is acceptable. This feature is critical, and is possible with the addition to the diet of supplements containing all of the essential amino acids as such or as their biochemical equivalents. Hence there is no need to be concerned about the amino acid composition of the foods consumed. This supplementation removes the threat of protein malnutrition, which has been the main argument against protein restriction.

In contrast, an unsupplemented low-protein diet, such as the 40 g protein diet that some nephrologists recommend (with the caveat that it may cause protein malnutrition) must emphasize so-called high-quality proteins, those proteins that contain very specific proportions of the essential amino acids. This requirement limits the variety of foods that can be included in the diet.

Another reason the very-low-protein diet is tolerated better than you might expect is because high-protein foods, such as meat and poultry, usually are totally excluded. For most patients (but not all), this is easier to adhere to than a diet that permits the occasional chicken or beef dish.

One reason these low-protein diets improve the signs and symptoms of renal failure is that they enable the body to utilize the nitrogen content of food more efficiently. You need less nitrogen in your diet to maintain your body's protein stores. Since intake of nitrogen seems to cause many of the signs and symptoms of kidney failure, less nitrogen makes people feel better.

If such diets slow the progression of kidney failure (which has not been firmly established, but is at least a possibility, as illustrated by a number of poorly controlled reports and by the case histories in Chapter 22), the mechanism by which they do so is unknown. One conceivable possibility is reduced cortisol production due to protein restriction; cortisol may play a role in disease progression.

One would suppose that a 40 g protein diet would be easier to follow than the one we recommend, but, in fact, the opposite is more often the case. In a study from Germany, patients reported a preference for the very-low-protein diet with supplements. A major difference, as explained earlier, is that there are no restrictions as to which foods are allowed, as long as they are low in protein.

In a random nine-month study, researchers compared a low-protein diet, limited to "high quality" proteins (the "potato-egg diet") with a diet containing 15 to 20 g of protein per day supplemented by essential amino acids. In patients on the supplemented diet, anemia was less severe, serum phosphorus levels were lower, and serum levels of several proteins were higher. The very-low-protein diet was thus more efficacious as well as easier to follow.

Taking Supplements with Your Diet

The very-low-protein diet requires not only supplements of essential amino acids (or their keto-analogues, which are converted in the body into the essential amino acids) but also supplemental vitamins and calcium, because very-low-protein diets usually contain inadequate amounts of these substances. Almost any multivitamin suffices, unless it contains added phosphate. However, vitamin requirements for those with advanced kidney failure are different. Specially formulated multivitamin preparations are available. (See Appendix 1.)

Calcium is best provided as calcium carbonate ($CaCO_3$), because other calcium salts, such as calcium lactate, contain substantially less calcium by weight. In other words, you need to take considerably larger doses to get the same amount of calcium. Calcium carbonate contains 40 percent calcium by weight, so to get 1,000 mg extra calcium daily, you would have to take 2,500 mg (2.5 g) of calcium carbonate. One easy way to achieve this is to take six Tums a day. To get the same amount of calcium as calcium lactate, for example, you would have to consume 5.5 g a day.

You may need extra zinc, too, because high-protein foods are the major source of zinc intake. Zinc gluconate is available in a 50 mg tablet, without a prescription.

Essential Amino Acid Supplements

The building blocks of protein are called amino acids. Proteins are composed of long chains of amino acids, with the chains folded in complex ways. Twenty different amino acids that are used in building proteins are known. Almost all of these 20 amino acids are found in almost all proteins, in differing sequences. These different sequences cause the chains to fold in different ways, bringing about myriad different functions. Of these 20 amino acids, 12 can be synthesized by the body from simpler constituents. The other 8 cannot; we must include them in our diet. For that reason these 8 are called essential amino acids. Just why the body cannot synthesize these amino acids remains a mystery. But all 8 of them are broken down at a slow rate.

In a series of experiments conducted over a 10-year period in the 1940s, Dr. William C. Rose determined the minimum requirements of each of the 8 essential amino acids by feeding subjects (students at the University of Illinois at Urbana) a protein-free diet supplemented by pure amino acids in varying quantities and measuring all nitrogen consumed (as food) and all nitrogen excreted (as urine plus stool). The difference between nitrogen intake and nitrogen output, called nitrogen balance, is a measure of change in total body protein. For each essential amino acid, intake below a certain amount led to negative nitrogen balance, indicating progressive loss of body protein stores, while intake above a certain amount led to positive nitrogen balance, showing that body protein stores were increasing. Just how Dr. Rose induced these students to consume what must have been a frightful diet, supplemented by unpleasant-tasting powders, remains a mystery, but this work stands as a landmark in the history of protein nutrition. Dr. Rose also demonstrated that most of the requirement for phenylalanine can be met by a closely related amino acid, tyrosine, and most of the requirement for methionine can be met by a closely related amino acid called cystine.

The quantities of each essential amino acid required for normal adults, in mg per kg per day, are held to be as follows, according to values given in *Recommended Dietary Allowances*, derived chiefly from Dr. Rose's work:

tryptophan	3.5
threonine	7
histidine	8 to 12
isoleucine	10
valine	10
lysine	12
methionine plus cystine	13
leucine	14
phenylalanine plus tyrosine	14

The total of these is 94 mg per kg per day, or 6.6 g per day (about 1½ teaspoonfuls) for a 70 kg (154 lb) person. Substantial caloric intake was necessary to achieve these results, and also a small amount of non-essential nitrogen from another nitrogen source, such as ammonium or glycine.

Thus, nutrition can be maintained on zero protein and as little as 10 g of amino acids, if a mixture of these 9 essential amino acids is provided and if calories, vitamins, and minerals are also provided in adequate amounts. This is nearly the diet that Giordano and Giovannetti gave to their patients. This approach has been a very unpopular because of the severely limited diet. The very-low-protein diet, supplemented by essential amino acids, is, by contrast, relatively acceptable. It contains little meat, poultry, fish, eggs, milk, or cheese, foods high in protein. But, if foods high in protein are avoided, the choice of foods is unlimited. The total dose of essential amino acids provided is usually 10 g per day, to be taken in three doses with meals. The reason for this recommendation is that it has been reported that nitrogen balance is better when all of the required amino acids are provided with a meal rather than between meals. The optimum dose is less certain.

The mixture of amino acids can be taken as a powder, mixed (for example) in apple sauce, but the taste is very unpleasant. More commonly it is taken as capsules or tablets. These tablets contain about 700 mg each, so the total daily dose is about 15 tablets.

Recently chemists have developed a way to mask the unpleasant taste of amino acids. Thus essential amino acids are available in almost any flavor as a powder that can be made into an instant beverage or candies. (See Appendix 1.)

These preparations, as well as pure amino acids, are considered dietary supplements and are therefore not subject to regulation by the Food and Drug Administration. The advantage is that they are readily available; the big disadvantage is that most insurers won't reimburse you for the cost. However, reimbursement for these products by Medicaid has been granted in several states.

Supplements of essential amino acids also improve nutrition (as evidenced by an increase in serum albumin levels, which reflect protein nutrition) in patients on hemodialysis, even without dietary protein restriction. Since they already are eating substantial amounts of protein, this is hard to explain. A randomized double-blind comparison study was performed on 29 patients on hemodialysis who had subnormal levels of serum albumin at the start. After three months, those on the amino acid supplement showed a significant increase in serum albumin concentration. The problem with this treatment was compliance: Patients grew tired of taking so many pills, and as the study progressed, they skipped more and more doses, or stopped taking supplements altogether. A parallel comparison in 18 patients on peritoneal dialysis failed to establish a significant effect on serum albumin level, perhaps because there were too few patients enrolled. Additional studies are in progress. It is hoped that the powder with the taste of amino acids masked may improve people's willingness to stick with the supplements.

Does Protein Restriction Cause Malnutrition?

One of the most tenacious misconceptions about kidney disease is the idea that increasing protein intake will improve protein nutrition. Logical though this seems, the opposite is more commonly the case.

Most patients with chronic kidney disease receive no dietary counseling and therefore make no change to their diets. For most Americans, this means a relatively high-protein diet. (We eat about twice as much protein as we need, on the average.) As the kidneys fail, products of protein breakdown progressively accumulate in the blood. Appetite falls off, and nausea and vomiting may occur. People consume fewer calories than they need, and malnutrition rears its head. Indeed, when dietary treatment is omitted, wasting develops sooner or later.

But any number of reports have documented that wasting is not a feature of properly treated kidney failure. In a paradox that has not been generally recognized, protein restriction *improves* protein nutrition.

When essential amino acids (or their keto-analogues) are given, protein intake can be severely restricted without inducing protein malnutrition. Indeed, this is exactly what Dr. Rose and his colleagues showed in normal college students many decades ago. Far from wasting, with the optimal mixture of amino acid supplements, but zero dietary protein, protein nutrition actually improved.

The largest study of protein nutrition in patients with kidney failure prescribed a very-low-protein diet was the Modification of Diet in Renal Disease (MDRD) study. As noted earlier, patients on such diets tend to reduce caloric intake at first, but as they get used to the diet, caloric intake recovers, and in the long term, nutrition is well maintained or even improves. Sophisticated markers of body composition may show significant declines during the first three months, but stabilize or improve thereafter.

I sincerely hope that as a patient with kidney failure, you give the very-low-protein diet supplemented with amino acids a try. I and many other researchers and doctors think that this diet will give you a fighting chance of slowing the course of your disease and delaying the need for you to go on dialysis.

8

Step 4: Treat Salt and Water Problems

One of the main jobs of the kidney is to regulate the salt (sodium chloride) and water content of the body, that is, the salt and water balance. It is not surprising, therefore, that patients with kidney disease have problems regulating the balance of salt and water, problems that become more troublesome as renal insufficiency gets more severe. In patients on dialysis, for example, who have little or no kidney function remaining, the regulation of salt and water balance becomes critical and must be watched very closely. Even people who have some residual kidney function are at risk to retain salt and water together (or separately; see below), which can cause the heart to fail.

Water Deficit without Salt Deficit

When the ratio of dissolved solids (mostly salt) to water gets over a certain limit, we feel thirsty and we find something to drink, thereby diluting the concentration of dissolved solids back down to the desired level. At the same time, the brain releases a hormone called vasopressin or anti-diuretic hormone that makes the kidney conserve water. But if there isn't much kidney function left, the organ can't respond to the hormone's chemical message. So although people with reduced kidney function can act on their thirst, they can't produce much concentrated urine.

Water Excess without Salt Excess

At the other extreme, when the concentration of dissolved solids gets below a certain limiting value, we lose all interest in drinking fluids. Our brains stop producing antidiuretic hormone. In the normal subject, this causes the urine to become very dilute and to increase enormously in volume. As a result, the concentration of dissolved solids returns to a normal value. In the subject with kidney disease, by contrast, there is little increase in urine flow and the urine doesn't become as dilute. Low concentration of dissolved solids is seen more commonly in patients with kidney disease than is high concentration of dissolved solids. This condition, when severe, is called water intoxication: its symptoms are variable, but often there is a severe headache.

Salt and Water Excess

Salt (sodium chloride) problems are much more prevalent in patients with kidney disease than water problems and are not as easy to treat. One reason is that humans don't have true salt hunger (or salt satiety), as many species of animals do. So we continue to consume salt (or to avoid it) whatever the needs of our body may be. By contrast, when we need water, we get thirsty.

Americans eat more salt than people in many societies, and it is particularly difficult for us to learn to eat foods without added salt. As the kidney is the only route for salt elimination, problems with salt retention are extremely common in patients with kidney disease. This is a universal problem in patients who have the nephrotic syndrome, as explained in Chapter 18. Salt retention always entails retention of a certain amount of water, as well, for reasons already explained: If you take salt with little or no water, you get thirsty because the concentration of dissolved solids in your body fluids has increased. Your brain releases antidiuretic hormone. These two responses result in increased intake of fluids and decreased excretion of urine, which together cause an increase in the amount of water in the body and a return to the normal level in the concentration of dissolved solids.

Salt and Water Deficit

Salt depletion is uncommon in chronic kidney disease, other than salt depletion caused by too vigorous use of diuretic drugs, as explained below. Some patients show a tendency to "waste" salt; that is, their kidneys (unlike normal kidneys) continue to excrete salt even when the body content is on the low side. But this defect is not likely to lead to symptomatic salt depletion unless dietary intake of salt is severely restricted and/or diuretic drugs are overused.

Hyponatremia (low serum sodium concentration) is much more common in patients with chronic renal failure than is hypernatremia (high serum sodium concentration). Hyponatremia in itself causes no symptoms unless it is severe. When patients drink too much water during their glomerular filtration rate (GFR) determination, they may develop very low serum sodium concentration, accompanied by severe headache and, rarely, by convulsions. This doesn't usually happen in people with normal or nearly normal kidney function because their bodies can increase their urine flow enough to get rid of the water load rapidly. They can, that is, unless they become nauseated or undergo a lot of pain during attempts at venipuncture. Both pain and nausea are powerful stimuli for the release of antidiuretic hormone, and can prevent the needed increase in urine flow. Hence, even normal people can suffer from hyponatremia during water loading for a GFR measurement, unless they are carefully instructed as to how much they should drink.

Occasionally people with chronic kidney disease may continuously drink more water than their kidneys can readily excrete and develop a serum sodium concentration low enough to be concerned about, say 126 mEq per liter or less. (The normal range is from 132 to 148 mEq per liter, but values between 126 and 132, even when maintained for years, don't seem to have any ill effects.) One reason people may drink so much is to relieve the dry mouth that a number of drugs, particularly drugs for hypertension, often produce.

Other individuals drink fluids compulsively. This is not connected with chronic kidney disease, except that the occurrence of both compulsive water drinking and chronic kidney disease in the same person makes hyponatremia very likely. This occurrence is greater than one would predict from chance alone, because neuropsychiatric disorders, including bipolar disorders and compulsive taking of laxatives, can both lead to the development of kidney disease (see Chapter 2), and compulsive water drinking can be associated with either of these disorders.

Rarely, a patient taking a thiazide diuretic (see below) may develop hyponatremia as a result of a direct action of the drug on the kidney, causing water retention—an action similar to that of vasopressin.

At the other extreme, if you lose salt without water for any reason, the concentration of dissolved solids in your body fluids becomes subnormal; thirst is turned off and usually vasopressin is turned off as well. The water content of the body diminishes and the concentration of dissolved solids returns to normal. All of these responses occur more rapidly in a normal subject than they do in a patient with chronic kidney disease, but even in such patients, they eventually result in water and salt balance changing together. Specifically, each 9 grams of salt retained (or lost) is accompanied by 1 liter (1 kg or 2.2 lb) of water. This is why measurement of the serum sodium concentration doesn't tell you anything about the amount of salt in the body; it measures something quite different, namely, the ratio of dissolved solids to water.

The Treatment of Hyponatremia

When pronounced hyponatremia develops (serum sodium concentration under, say, 125 mEq per liter) and persists more than overnight, it is worth treating by the simple measure of fluid restriction. The reason this works, albeit slowly, is that water loss by evaporation through the skin continues no matter what, at a rate of about a liter a day. So serum sodium concentration gradually comes up to normal. It is often sufficient merely to tell the patient to cut down on fluids, rather than to limit intake to some measured amount.

Edema

When salt (and water) are retained, the result is edema, which means swelling of the soft tissues from fluid. The fluid accumulates by gravity in the lowest part of the body; at night, this means the back, where it is seldom noticed. In the daytime it appears in the ankles and feet most noticeably, particularly at the end of the day. It is detected by pressing the body with a finger or thumb for a few seconds and then releasing; a dent remains. This is called "pitting edema." Other parts of the body may swell, too. For example, some patients (women in particular, I think) notice swelling of the abdomen even when there is no pitting edema. When fluid accumulates within the air spaces of the lungs (pulmonary edema), exchanges of oxygen and carbon dioxide are impaired; as a result, the heart may fail. Pulmonary edema is a medical emergency.

Although edema is rather uncomfortable, in itself it is not serious unless it occurs in the lungs. A small amount of edema may in fact be desirable in many patients, because when they take diuretics to remove the excess fluid, their blood pressure falls too far. The problem is that the associated increase in the volume of body fluids often aggravates hypertension and/or congestive heart failure in patients suffering from these complications. Both of these conditions are acutely sensitive to the volume of the extracellular fluids.

Treatment of edema is usually straightforward, except in the nephrotic syndrome. (See Chapter 18.) Restriction of salt intake plus administration of diuretic drugs generally does the trick. That said, it is foolish to give diuretic drugs without some attempt to restrict salt intake, because doing so would be self-defeating. However, severe salt restriction is not advisable because it is so unpalatable. In order to limit salt intake moderately, simply refrain from adding salt to food during cooking and at the table. Also avoid prepared foods high in sodium, as indicated by nutrition labels.

Diuretics

Diuretics, which are probably the most widely prescribed drugs (next to birth control pills), increase the kidneys' output of salt and water. They are used for two main purposes: to reduce salt and water accumulation and to reduce blood pressure. The first effect tends to reduce blood pressure by itself, but some of these drugs also have a direct effect on blood pressure, by dilating blood vessels.

One of the most widely used classes of diuretic drugs, the loop diuretics, markedly inhibit salt reabsorption by the kidney tubules. They are very effective, even in severe kidney failure, even though it may be necessary to increase the dose substantially beyond the usually recommended doses. Fortunately these drugs have very low toxicity. One of the most commonly used drugs of this class is furosemide. It is best given twice a day, because with a single dose there is rebound salt retention in the other 12 hours of the day. Giving it at night probably will increase nocturnal voiding, but this is a price that must be paid. The usual starting dose is 20 to 40 mg twice a day. It can be increased safely to at least 200 mg twice a day in cases of severe kidney failure. Occasionally hearing may become impaired at higher doses. If the drug is stopped, hearing generally returns to normal, but a very small number of patients develop permanent partial or even complete hearing loss. Large doses also may cause nausea and vomiting, but in my experience, this is seen only after intravenous administration.

Loop diuretics tend to cause increased loss of potassium in the urine and occasionally can cause potassium deficiency, as discussed further in Chapter 12. They also may increase serum uric acid and may precipitate gout, as discussed in Chapter 14.

If loop diuretics alone don't do the trick, the addition of a thiazide diuretic like metolazone will, in most cases. In fact, the main problem with this combination is that it may be too effective.

Can diuresis be overdone? The answer is an emphatic yes. Too much diuresis triggers a set of reflex responses that may have devastating effects in patients with kidney failure. The most prominent feature of this response is a decrease in the blood flow to the kidneys. GFR falls sharply, too. In fact, blood flow to the kidneys is decreased more than blood flow to any other organ. This protective response is very useful in normal subjects. When the volume of body fluids is restored, their kidney blood flow and GFR return to normal. In patients with kidney failure, by contrast, recovery of blood flow and GFR may be limited or may not occur at all.

Under these circumstances of reduced body fluid volume, the brain releases vasopressin in an attempt to restore volume, even though water retention cannot make up for a salt deficit. As a result, hyponatremia occurs. This is the one form of hyponatremia in which a low serum sodium concentration is associated with a sodium deficit. Treatment for this condition, which has the wordy name syndrome of inappropriate antidiuretic hormone secretion, is fluid restriction plus liberalization of salt intake.

Thiazide diuretics also can be used alone. Formerly these drugs were not recommended in patients with kidney failure because they tend to cause an acute drop in GFR when first administered. However, this drop is small and does not mean that GFR will continue to fall. The main advantage of thiazide diuretics is that they have a direct effect of lowering blood pressure. They are also the least expensive diuretics available. However, they do cause more potassium loss than loop diuretics, and this may become a problem. (See Chapter 12.) It is advisable for your doctor to check serum potassium after a couple of weeks and then at infrequent intervals. Thiazide diuretics also may aggravate elevations of serum cholesterol and triglycerides (see Chapter 15), and uric acid accumulation (see Chapter 14) and may increase insulin requirements in patients with diabetes. All of these side effects, however, are dose-dependent and are uncommon at low dosage.

Other classes of diuretic drugs are not usually recommended for patients with kidney failure, either because they are not very effective or because of side effects. Potassium-sparing diuretics, such as amiloride, triamterene, and spironolactone, should not be used as the sole diuretic in patients with moderate or severe chronic renal failure because of the danger of potassium retention. (See Chapter 12.)

Judging Your Salt and Water Balance

How can you judge the optimal volume of extracellular fluids, in other words, the optimal body content of salt and water? The best way I know is to measure your blood pressure in both prone and sitting (or standing) positions. Normally, blood pressure rises when we sit or stand. When the volume of extracellular fluids is too low, it falls instead. This fall in blood pressure may cause what are called "orthostatic" symptoms, namely, faintness, dizziness, or blacking out on standing up.

If these signs or symptoms are seen while edema is still present, the edema is not only desirable but necessary in order to achieve an adequate blood flow to the kidneys. Continuing diuretic drug treatment until "dry weight" has been achieved is likely to lower GFR and hasten dialysis.

Enlargement and thickening of the left ventricle of the heart (left ventricular hypertrophy) is common in patients with renal failure, partly because hypertension is so common, and it increases the work of the heart; another factor is anemia, which also means that the heart must work harder to get enough oxygen to the tissues. Abnormalities of the heart's pump function are seen in most patients with kidney failure. Digoxin and related drugs, which often are used to treat heart failure in subjects without kidney disease, should probably be avoided, because the symptoms of toxicity from these drugs are so similar to the symptoms of renal failure. Diuretics, angiotensin-converting-enzyme inhibitors, and angiotensin receptor blockers may be useful. When heart failure becomes pronounced despite these measures, the only alternative may be dialysis, even though such patients do not do well on dialysis.

9

Step 5: Regulate Your Blood Pressure

The next step in taking control of your kidney health is to regulate your blood pressure. Doctors call high blood pressure the silent killer, because most people feel no symptoms, except an occasional headache. High blood pressure can exist for decades before being detected. Yet it can cause serious damage. It's the leading cause of heart disease and strokes. It also can cause damage to the eyes and kidneys, as detailed later. The malignant kind, which is especially severe and is accompanied by swelling of the optic nerve head in the retina, can lead rapidly to kidney failure. It is also clear that, in people who already have some loss of kidney function for any reason, lowering blood pressure will slow the rate of further damage. Before we get to why it's important to pay attention to blood pressure, let's first take a brief look at what blood pressure is.

What Is Blood Pressure?

The circulation of the blood provides nourishment to the trillions of cells that make up our bodies. Blood carries oxygen, sugars, proteins, and hundreds of foodstuffs throughout the body. About a gallon of blood does the job. But it has to be pumped through the blood vessels, some 60,000 miles of them, in fact. To do this some blood pressure is essential. The heart is a pulsing muscle that squeezes blood in and out some 70 times a minute, creating pressure in the arteries. The largest artery, called the aorta, serves as the main channel for blood leaving the heart. The aorta branches into smaller arteries, which in turn branch into smaller arteries called arterioles. As these branch into smaller and smaller tubes, they end up in tiny capillaries, barely wide enough to permit the passage of a single red blood cell at a time. Across the walls of these capillaries, oxygen and nutrients diffuse into the tissues, while waste products and carbon dioxide diffuse from the tissues into the capillaries. Then the capillaries drain into veins, which are tiny at first, but get bigger and bigger as they approach the heart. When blood from the veins reaches your heart, it is pumped to your lungs, where it releases carbon dioxide and picks up a new supply of oxygen. This blood is then sent back to your heart to start over again. Meanwhile the kidneys excrete waste products.

Blood pressure varies throughout the day. When you sleep, blood pressure falls; your tissues need less oxygen and nutrients. When you exercise, the opposite happens. Your muscles need more oxygen and energy to perform work, and your blood pressure rises, increasing blood flow to the tissues that need it most. Even standing up affects blood pressure: To get more blood up to your brain, blood pressure rises.

Your body controls blood pressure in two ways: by changes in the rate and force of contraction of the heart in response to nerve impulses from the brain, and by changes in the blood flow through small arteries. When these arteries constrict, more pressure is required to achieve the same flow; when the small arteries relax, blood pressure falls.

The control mechanism for these amazing responses includes detectors called baroreceptors, found in the large arteries in the neck and in the kidneys. These detectors are attuned to pressure and exert their effects in two ways:

1. By sending nerve impulses that signal the heart to increase the rate and force of the heart muscle contractions.

2. By affecting the production of several hormones. The first of these is renin, made mainly in the kidneys. Renin reacts with a second hormone called angiotensinogen, produced in the liver, to form angiotensin I. This is not very active itself, but when your blood

carries angiotensin I to your lungs, it's converted to angiotensin II, a very potent constrictor of blood vessels. Angiotensin II also stimulates the adrenal cortex to produce yet another hormone, called aldosterone. This steroid hormone, closely related to cortisol, plays a major role in stimulating the kidney to excrete potassium and to retain sodium. In fact, in its absence, the body may retain potassium to a dangerous degree. (See Chapter 12.) But we now know that aldosterone also exerts a number of harmful effects, especially on the heart. This curious set of circumstances complicates treatment.

A major determinant of blood pressure is salt intake. Salt intake affects blood pressure primarily by altering the volume of body fluids. Even in a healthy person, a high salt intake (say, 15 g per day) is associated with a roughly 7-pound higher weight, owing to more fluid between the cells. There is also some difference in blood pressure. The person with a higher salt intake usually has a higher blood pressure, a fact explained most simply by postulating that it takes more pressure to force the greater blood volume through the blood vessels.

People with high blood pressure vary dramatically in their sensitivity to salt. Some show big changes in blood pressure with minor changes in salt intake; others do not. Older people, African Americans, and those with family histories of hypertension will experience the biggest drop in blood pressure when they limit their salt intake.

High Blood Pressure and Kidney Failure

Hypertension (high blood pressure) is a common feature of renal failure. It appears in most patients at some point as the disease progresses. The reasons for hypertension in almost all patients with chronic kidney disease (in addition to those whose hypertension is their primary disorder) are complex, but have to do with hormones produced by normal kidneys that regulate blood pressure, especially hormones that control sodium balance. In susceptible people, retention of sodium increases blood pressure, and hormones that increase the sodium content of the body tend to be produced in increased amounts. Other hormones may play a role in hypertension as well, including parathyroid hormone and insulin, both of which tend to rise in patients with hypertension. The body tends to produce decreased amounts of substances normally released by the kidneys that lower blood pressure. For these many reasons, high blood pressure is a very common feature of kidney failure.

Occasionally people have high blood pressure caused by the narrowing of one or both of the arteries that lead to the kidneys. Many of these patients can be cured surgically, especially if only one kidney is involved.

Because hypertension further damages diseased kidneys, albeit slowly, it is important to control it. There is a rather clear-cut relationship between blood pressure and the rate of progression of kidney failure, at least in certain subgroups (particularly in those with substantial amounts of protein in their urine—for example, more than 4 g per day.) People with diabetes and kidney disease progress more rapidly if their systolic blood pressure is high; diastolic blood pressure is a weaker predictor. Reduction of systolic blood pressure by giving an angiotensin receptor blocker slows disease progression.

Treating High Blood Pressure

High blood pressure can be treated, either by lifestyle changes such as diet, exercise, and smoking cessation, or, if necessary, by drugs. Diet changes that are particularly effective in lowering blood pressure include restricting your consumption of calories and salt, eating more vegetables and fruits, and reading food labels closely so as to limit intake of sodium and of saturated fats.

First, you may need to lose weight. "Ideal" body weights for men and women of varying heights and frame size are available elsewhere. (For example, see Appendix 9 of *Nutritional Management*; for the full citation, see Appendix 1 of this book.) To determine your frame size, measure your wrist circumference by placing a soft measuring tape around the smallest part of the wrist. The ratio of your height to your wrist circumference (in inches or whatever units you prefer) is an index of your frame size. Use this table to see if your frame is small, medium, or large.

Frame	Men	Women
Small	10.4	11.1
Medium	9.7–10.3	10.2–11.0
Large	9.6	10.1

Based on your frame size, you may learn that you exceed your "ideal" weight. If so, don't be alarmed. Most Americans exceed that weight. There's no need to achieve model thinness, because losing just a few pounds can have substantial medical benefits. Losing as few as 10 pounds can drop your blood pressure by about 7 points. This alone can mean the difference between hypertension and high-normal blood pressure. Loss of a pound or two a week is about right. "Crash" diets that promise you'll lose weight faster usually have only temporary benefits; the weight comes back. Diets rich in fruits and vegetables can be extraordinarily effective in lowering blood pressure, partly because they are rich in potassium, which counteracts sodium's effect on blood pressure.

Even if you don't have hypertension, losing a few pounds may help keep your blood pressure in the normal range.

Sodium, one of the ingredients of sodium chloride (table salt), plays a major role in hypertension. As mentioned, Americans in particular eat far too much salt. Meat, cheese, cereal, soups, pretzels, potato chips, tuna, bread, spaghetti sauce, and many other foods are salt-rich American favorites. We eat an average of 25 times as much as we need, because we like it. The salt content of processed foods is particularly high, especially canned or packaged products. Breads and cereals provide almost one-third of the salt we eat.

Rarely, people who tend to faint a lot could make things worse but cutting down on salt. If you think you might have this problem, talk to your doctor.

Measuring Your Own Blood Pressure

All patients with kidney disease should learn to measure their own blood pressure in the arm; how often they need to take the measurement depends on whether it is high or not; if it is normal, check it at least once a month to make sure it stays that way. If you have high blood pressure, check it and record it at least once a week, at about the same time of day. Show your blood presssure log to your doctor. If your blood pressure is consistently elevated, or if protein is consistently in your urine, see your doctor.

Devices for self-measurement of blood pressure are available without a prescription at any drugstore. Buy the less expensive variety, with a stethoscope attached, rather than the more expensive electronic variety.

Learning to use a stethoscope takes a bit of practice, but the digital readout device is somewhat less reliable. If you can't master the self-measurement of blood pressure with a stethoscope, get an electronic device. In 1996, *Consumer Reports* rated 16 makes.

The best way to measure blood pressure is with an inflatable cuff on the upper arm (either arm) and a stethoscope. Inflate the cuff (which must be firmly placed; subjects who are very large should use a larger cuff known as a thigh cuff, placed high on the arm) to a pressure over 200 mm mercury or so, and then gradually deflate it so that the pressure in the cuff falls about 10 mm every two seconds or so, as indicated on the device. When you reach the systolic pressure you will hear a sound through the stethoscope with every heartbeat. Continue to lower the pressure at the same rate. Eventually the sounds will disappear. The pressure at which the sounds disappear is the diastolic blood pressure.

It is important to place the diaphragm of the stethoscope right over the brachial artery. You can locate this spot in the crease of your elbow by feeling there for a pulse. If you place the stethoscope incorrectly, you may not hear anything. There may be variation between beats in both the systolic and the diastolic pressure, particularly if your heart rate is irregular for any reason. Under these conditions, there is necessarily a degree of arbitrariness in deciding exactly what is the systolic and the diastolic pressure. In some individuals, the brachial pulse is not pronounced and it may be very hard to hear anything, even when the stethoscope is placed correctly.

Why measure your own blood pressure? Well, blood pressures measured by patients themselves are often more informative than those measured in the office, for two reasons: (1) water loading for a glomerular filtration rate test increases blood pressure; (2) visiting the doctor's office is anxiety-producing and raises blood pressure. The average of many values recorded by the patient, if accurately measured, gives a much better idea of long-term blood pressure control than does a single value recorded at an office visit.

Current recommendations are to keep mean arterial blood pressure (systolic pressure plus two times diastolic pressure, divided by three) under 95 mm Hg in patients with renal failure. This is lower than has been recommended in the past. A blood pressure of 130/80, for example, signifies a mean arterial pressure of 97 mm Hg and is slightly high. Pronounced hypertension (say, over 160/100) can not only damage the kidney but also can lead to strokes, visual disorders, and heart failure, and must be treated urgently. According to recent information, systolic blood pressure is much more important than diastolic blood pressure.

If you have high blood pressure, check it and record it at least once a week, at about the same time of day. Show your blood pressure log to your doctor. If your blood pressure is consistently elevated, or if protein is consistently in your urine, see your doctor.

As noted earlier, there is a strong relationship between hypertension and salt balance, and this relationship is even stronger in the presence of kidney failure. Many patients will present with hypertension accompanied by signs of fluid retention; when appropriate diuresis (excretion of salt and water excess) is achieved, the blood pressure may return to normal. It follows that control of salt balance should be a first priority in treating hypertension in patients with kidney disease, and that variations in blood pressure associated with and caused by salt and water retention are best treated with salt restriction and diuretic drugs, as described in the preceding section.

But achieving an optimal extracellular fluid volume often does not bring blood pressure back to normal. Most patients will require antihypertensive drugs, commonly in combination.

Medications for High Blood Pressure

Before getting into specifics about drug treatment of high blood pressure in people with kidney disease, I want to emphasize some general principles.

- The lowest effective dose should always be used. It is necessary to start on a dose that will not be fully effective and to increase the dose gradually until you reach the lowest effective dose. Antihypertensive drugs all cause dose-dependent adverse effects, and unfortunately they often are prescribed in doses higher than necessary.
- The ideal is a slow fall in blood pressure, not a rapid one. With a rapid fall in blood pressure, you may notice signs of reduced blood flow to the brain, such as weakness, fatigue, and dizziness on standing.
- The goal is to reduce blood pressure throughout the 24-hour period. Taking your drugs at bedtime is not a good idea; you need to control

your blood pressure in the daytime, as well, so take them in the morning.

- Treatment works only if you take the prescribed medications. Research has found that only half of people with high blood pressure continue their medications after a few months. Just why this is so is uncertain. Part of the reason is because of side effects, which are numerous, but some people seem to quit for no apparent reason.

- Blood pressure varies a good deal from day to day and in the course of a single day. Highest pressure is usually in the late afternoon. Measure your blood pressure at about the same time every day. How often you record it depends on the severity of hypertension, but I have found that patients who measure blood pressure every day have less difficulty in remembering to do it. Although devices are now available that measure blood pressure automatically and record it every 20 minutes or so, around the clock, most patients don't need to use these expensive devices.

Drug treatment of high blood pressure in people with kidney disease is not the same as drug treatment of people who have high blood pressure without kidney failure. Nevertheless, the categories of drugs that are used are the same:

- Diuretics
- Adrenergic inhibitors which block the formation or action of a group of hormones, including adrenaline (epinephrine), that tend to raise blood pressure
- Angiotensin inhibitors and angiotensin receptor blockers
- Calcium channel blockers
- Direct vasodilators

Individual drugs in these categories are employed differently. It is usually necessary to use at least two drugs, selecting agents from at least two different categories.

Diuretics

Diuretics are drugs that increase salt excretion by the kidneys. As discussed earlier, there is a strong relationship between blood pressure and body salt content; hence drugs that diminish body salt content tend to lower blood pressure. Dietary salt restriction should be tried first, since giving a diuretic to a subject consuming a high salt intake is folly. As discussed in Chapter 8, I recommend moderate restriction of salt intake in almost all my patients. This includes avoiding foods with high sodium content (such as most packaged foods) and avoiding added salt in cooking or at the table. More severe salt restriction makes food very unpalatable, and caloric intake may decrease. The rare patient has a tendency to lose salt and can become salt-depleted easily.

The most widely employed class of diuretics, thiazide diuretics, are not very powerful as antihypertensive drugs. Not many patients' blood pressure can be controlled with a thiazide alone, unless their only problem is salt and water retention. The antihypertensive effect of thiazides may take several weeks to become fully expressed, long after the loss of salt and water has occurred. Clearly thiazides lower blood pressure by more than one mechanism.

In people with diabetes, thiazides (especially in substantial doses) may increase insulin requirements. They also may aggravate lipid disorders (see Chapter 15) and cause substantial potassium loss. This potassium loss can cause serious heart rhythm disturbances if it is not recognized and treated (see Chapter 12) and may precipitate attacks of gout (see Chapter 14). As noted earlier, however, all of these side effects are dose-dependent and not commonly seen on low doses, which are often enough for the treatment of hypertension. A dose of 12.5 mg per day of hydrochlorothiazide is usually about right, even though no such tablet can be purchased. If you're prescribed this dose, you'll be buying 25 mg tablets and breaking them in half.

Chlorthalidone, another thiazide, recently has been shown to be particularly effective in preventing heart failure, at least in people without kidney disease.

Adrenergic Inhibitors

The most widely used subgroup of these drugs are the so called beta-blockers, meaning that these drugs block a certain group of receptors in the sympathetic nervous system. Atenolol and metoprolol are two of these drugs. They not only lower blood pressure but also slow heart rate, and therefore are particularly useful in conjunction with other drugs that tend to increase heart rate. They do, however, have a huge variety of side effects, which can be troublesome. Alpha-blockers, such as doxazosin and terazosin, which block a different set of sympathetic receptors and do not tend to slow the heart, are also available, and also lower blood pressure.

Angiotensin-Converting Enzyme Inhibitors and Angiotensin Receptor Blockers

Angiotensin-converting enzyme inhibitors (ACEIs) and angiotensin receptor blockers (ARBs) inhibit the formation or action of angiotensin and are very effective in the treatment of hypertension.

ACEIs cause a persistent chronic cough in many patients, which often goes undiagnosed for months; ARBs apparently do not have this effect. The most serious limitation of these two classes of drugs, however, is that they cause potassium retention. As noted in Chapter 12, this is more insidious than potassium deficiency, because there are few if any symptoms associated with potassium excess, which can cause sudden death; it is frequently undiagnosed. Unlike other classes of antihypertensive drugs, these drugs specifically slow the progression of kidney disease by a small but significant amount, above and beyond their effect to lower blood pressure.

As noted earlier, ARBs slow progression of diabetic nephropathy.

Calcium Channel Blockers

Calcium channel blockers, relatively new agents, inhibit the passage of nerve impulses through cell membranes. This seems to lower blood pressure quite effectively.

Direct Vasodilators

Drugs classed as direct vasodilators include hydralazine and minoxidil, which act directly on blood vessels.

Unfortunately, all of these drugs have multitudinous side effects, which are often troublesome. In particular, salt and water retention is prominent with calcium channel blockers like nifedipine. Minoxidil causes even more severe salt and water retention; in addition, it makes hair grow (including on the head, which is why it is now marketed as an ointment, Rogaine); this is not troublesome to most men, but can be very distressing in women.

10

Step 6:
Treat Acidosis

A condition called acidosis may be causing you fatigue and malaise and also may be preventing your body from being properly nourished. It also may be aggravating some of your symptoms of kidney failure. Happily, the cure for this condition is very easy. Let's take a quick look at what acidosis is before I describe the treatment for it.

Acidosis

Blood is normally slightly alkaline. Two mechanisms regulate its level of acidity-alkalinity: (1) the rate of breathing (which determines the rate at which carbon dioxide, produced continuously by metabolism, is exhaled), and (2) the kidneys, which regulate the rate of excretion of acid, or when necessary, of alkali (as sodium bicarbonate).

Acidosis is the name for a relatively acid condition of the extracellular fluid (blood and the fluid between cells). It occurs with great frequency in kidney failure, because the kidneys fail to retain alkaline bicarbonate. The resulting acidosis tends to cause protein wasting and may cause fatigue.

Alkalosis

Alkalosis is the name for an abnormally alkaline condition of the extra-cellular fluid. Occasionally subjects (with or without kidney failure) breathe too rapidly, generally because of anxiety, and they exhale so much carbon dioxide that the CO_2 level in body fluids falls. Generally there is no difficulty recognizing this disorder and distinguishing it from the much more common cause of low CO_2, namely, acidosis. The usual treatment of hyperventilation alkalosis is to get the patient to breathe into a paper bag, where CO_2 accumulates. As the patient begins to inhale a greater concentration of CO_2, the CO_2 level of body fluids is restored and the alkalosis is corrected. The symptoms of alkalosis, namely numbness and tingling around the mouth, muscle cramps, and worsening anxiety, subside as the alkalosis is corrected.

The easiest way to ascertain a person's acid-base status is to measure the concentration of bicarbonate in the plasma or serum. Bicarbonate is alkaline, and the lower its concentration, the more acidic the body fluids are likely to be. A normal concentration is about 24 mM. In patients with kidney disease, the kidneys often spill bicarbonate into the urine even when it is not present in excess amounts in the blood; as a result, its concentration in the plasma or serum often falls below normal, resulting in acidosis.

Treatment

There is no excuse for uncorrected acidosis, because the treatment is extremely simple and effective. Oral sodium bicarbonate tablets, taken daily, completely correct it. These are sold, without a prescription, as 10 grain tablets (1 grain = 65 mg). Sometimes they are called bicarb of soda. You probably have some in the kitchen cabinet in its powder form (Arm & Hammer Baking Soda®), but don't take it; it tastes pretty bad.

Why this archaic grain unit is still used for sodium bicarbonate is a mystery. The required dose, which your doctor will specify, varies from 3 to 8 tablets a day. There are no side effects and no toxicity, except that ingestion of the tablets causes belching or sometimes flatus. You can take the tablets all at once or spaced throughout the day.

Some nephrologists continue to ignore all but the most severe acidosis in patients with renal failure, maintaining that treatment is unnecessary. To my thinking, this view is indefensible. Why not treat an abnormality, if it can be done easily and cheaply, and might help?

Some physicians claim that they cannot give enough sodium bicarbonate to treat or prevent acidosis because of the resulting sodium retention. But increasing the dose of an effective diuretic, such as furosemide or furosemide plus metolazone, will get rid of any retained sodium.

Alkalosis, or high bicarbonate levels, is also seen in renal failure, reflecting a defect in acid-base regulation. As far as I know, it has no adverse consequences and no treatment is required.

11

Step 7: Treat Anemia and Iron Deficiency

Anemia, or low red cell count, low hemoglobin concentration, and low hematocrit, is seen sooner or later in many cases of renal failure. Anemia occurs in patients with kidney failure because the hormone that signals the bone marrow to produce more red cells, erythropoietin, is synthesized in the kidney, and this process may be inadequate in people with kidney disease. Anemia in patients with chronic renal failure may cause shortness of breath on exertion and even frank heart failure. Anemia severe enough to cause symptoms is seen in about one-third of patients.

Treatment

When symptomatic, anemia generally is treated with erythropoietin injections (Epogen or Procrit). Quality of life may improve after treatment. In fact, treatment may be useful even if there are no specific symptoms, because patients may experience increased strength and vigor.

Your doctor may aim to increase your hematocrit to no more than 36 percent or so (instead of all the way up to normal, that is, about 40 percent) because aggravating hypertension becomes a problem as a normal level of hematocrit is approached. At first, there was concern that treatment with erythropoietin might accelerate the progression of chronic renal failure. This turns out not to be the case; in fact, some authors report that progression slows with such treatment.

Iron Deficiency

Iron deficiency also is seen in about a third of predialysis patients, whether anemia is present or not, but is even more common in patients who have been given erythropoietin injections. This results because their bone marrow is stimulated to produce extra hemoglobin, which contains iron; as a result, their iron stores become depleted.

There are several blood tests for assessing iron stores, including serum iron, serum ferritin, serum iron-binding protein, and the level of this protein's saturation with iron. We have relied chiefly on serum iron determinations, which are not infrequently subnormal in patients with renal failure. Surprisingly, we have found that there is a correlation between iron concentration in the serum and albumin concentration. In other words, patients who are relatively less well nourished also have relatively low serum iron levels. Patients who have the nephrotic syndrome (see Chapter 18), with much lower serum albumin levels, also had very low serum iron levels; this is probably explained by the well-known observation that urinary iron excretion is markedly increased in the nephrotic syndrome. Urinary iron excretion is also increased early in the course of diabetic renal disease, which may be a factor in causing iron deficiency. It remains to be proven that iron supplementation improves serum albumin level, although it might. If you are iron deficient, it is certainly worth treating.

Treatment of Iron Deficiency

When iron deficiency is diagnosed, its treatment is generally simple: oral tablets of ferrous sulfate. These tablets are usually 325 mg each, and the required dose may be from one to three tablets daily. Unfortunately, digestive disturbances such as diarrhea, constipation, or gastric distress are common. Many other iron preparations are on the market, all of which claim to cause fewer digestive symptoms. In some patients, these other preparations may indeed be less troublesome.

Another problem with iron supplementation is that the stools become black or blackish green. This result is not dangerous and is not to be confused with tarry and sticky black stools caused by upper gastrointestinal hemorrhage. However, some patients may find the change disturbing.

For some patients iron supplements are ineffective. We do not know why some people fail to absorb supplementary iron. These patients may require intravenous iron. The kind of intravenous iron formerly used in the United States, iron dextran, caused death in approximately 0.7 percent of patients due to allergic reactions, making its use very dubious; however, iron sucrose, which has been used safely in Europe for decades, is now available here. So is ferric gluconate, another form of intravenous iron.

Recently, the effectiveness of iron sucrose, given intravenously weekly for five weeks, was compared with the same treatment plus erythropoietin injections in 90 anemic predialysis patients. Hematocrit rose rapidly in both groups and often could be maintained with iron treatments alone.

12

Step 8: Treat Potassium Problems

Potassium, like sodium, is one of the main minerals of the body. Unlike sodium, it is found chiefly within cells rather than between them. It plays a critical role in muscular contraction, especially in the heart.

There are two problems with potassium levels among patients with chronic renal failure. One is too little, and the other is too much (medically known as hyperkaliemia). Excessive potassium is a much more common and dangerous problem than potassium deficiency, so let's look at it first.

Excessive Potassium

Excess potassium leads to an increase in serum potassium concentration above the upper limit of normal, a condition called hyperkaliemia. Normal serum potassium concentration is 3 to 5 mEq per liter. At 5 to 6 mEq per liter, hyperkaliemia is not threatening, but above 6 mEq per liter, it is very dangerous. Occasional patients may develop intestinal symptoms, but generally hyperkaliemia causes no symptoms. Sudden death from cardiac arrest occurs without warning. The electrocardiogram will show signs of hyperkaliemia, but usually one is not ordered because the patient presents no clinical signs of heart problems. Sometimes there is accompanying acidosis.

Nowadays the most common cause of hyperkaliemia in chronic renal failure is drugs, namely angiotensin-converting enzyme inhibitors (ACEIs) or angiotensin receptor blockers (ARBs). (See Chapters 9 and 12.) These drugs inhibit angiotensin formation or action. Angiotensin is the main stimulus to the production of aldosterone, a hormone that promotes potassium excretion. Unless aldosterone secretion increases and promotes potassium excretion, potassium may accumulate in the body. As renal failure becomes more severe, the dangers of these drugs increase. If you're on one of these drugs, your physician should monitor serum potassium about once a month.

Unfortunately, that's far from current practice. In a recent study, *every one* of patients with chronic renal failure on ACEIs who had severe kidney disease, as shown by a serum creatinine level of 4 mg per dl or higher, also had hyperkaliemia. A substantial number of patients with less severe renal failure or even with normal renal function (as shown by their serum creatinine levels) also had hyperkaliemia. In one-third of the 119 patients, ACEIs had to be withdrawn, after dose reduction and dietary potassium restriction had failed to control the problem. The authors of the study could not determine how many patients had died of hyperkaliemia, although they cited several references to fatal cases. There is no evidence upon autopsy of hyperkaliemia in patients who die of excessive potassium. How can we determine how often ACEIs cause death? Unfortunately, we cannot. I personally do not recommend ACEIs and ARBs for patients with severe renal failure. This view is the opposite of current opinion, which calls these drugs renoprotective and panaceas. In fact, the *Physicians' Desk Reference (PDR)* scarcely mentions the dangers of hyperkaliemia with these drugs, nor do their main advocates. This is probably because advocates of these drugs did not treat many patients with severe renal failure. (For further information see my letter published in the *New England Journal of Medicine* 346: 706, 2002, and the replies to it.)

Another cause of hyperkaliemia is the use of diuretic drugs that promote potassium retention, such as triamterene, amiloride, and spironolactone. Generally these "potassium-sparing" diuretics should not be prescribed in patients with moderate or severe renal failure.

Finally, there are patients who develop hyperkaliemia apparently because of a defect in adrenal/renal regulation of potassium balance.

Albert Prendergass,a 22-year-old college student from Annapolis,was referred to Johns Hopkins by an Annapolis physician. He had had kidney disease since the age of 14, when he developed ankle and facial swelling, fatigue, and severe hypertension. A kidney biopsy showed glomerulonephritis. A course of prednisone therapy didn't help. For several years he had taken a variety of antihypertensive medications, including captopril, an ACE inhibitor. Serum creatinine concentration was first noted to be elevated (to 2.1 mg per /dl) three years ago. He has recently developed muscle cramps, headaches, and loss of appetite. A few hours after he left the clinic, the lab called with a "panic" value: serum potassium 7.6 mEq per liter, close to the level at which cardiac arrest occurs. Serum creatinine was 7.9 mg per dl. Albert had left no phone number because he didn't have a phone. He had left a work number, but it was by now after hours. I recalled that he had said that his parents lived somewhere in northern California. With the help of a telephone operator, I found them and told them that I needed to reach their son urgently. They gave me the number of his college and eventually, I got him out of an evening class and told to to go immediately to the drugstore, where I called in a prescription for sodium polystyrene sulfonate (SPS). He took the drug and, within a week, his serum potassium had fallen to 6 mEq per liter and within three weeks to normal (4.8 mEq per liter). His renal failure was too severe to treat with nutritional therapy, and he soon went on dialysis.

Clearly, Albert had developed hyperkaliemia as a result of taking of an ACE inhibitor. Had he not shown up by chance when he did, he might have died of cardiac arrest. Although his physician had followed his serum creatinine levels, that wasn't enough.

Treatment of Excessive Potassium

The treatment of hyperkaliemia is usually not difficult. If it is extreme (greater than 6.5 mEq per liter), urgent treatment is indicated. Therapy may include intravenous glucose and insulin, intravenous calcium salts, or albuterol inhalation. If these measures are inadequate, it may be necessary to initiate dialysis. In less urgent cases, sodium polystyrene sulfonate, an exchange resin taken in the sodium form that is not absorbed in the intestine, but takes up potassium in exchange for sodium and is excreted in the stool, can be taken by mouth. This drug is expensive and difficult to take. (It tastes like sand.) It is usually dispensed in sorbitol suspension so as to reduce its constipating effects. However, in some patients the sorbitol leads to diarrhea or to more serious intestinal problems. Other laxatives may be safer and may in fact lower potassium somewhat when given alone (that is, without the SPS). SPS without sorbitol is also available (Kionex). In mild cases, reduction of dietary potassium also may help, though in my opinion that idea is a nonstarter. I never use this last option because small doses of SPS are so effective and these patients already struggle with a multitude of dietary restrictions. If there is associated acidosis and the hyperkalemia is mild, sodium bicarbonate (see Chapter 10) can address both problems.

Twenty percent of my patients on the very-low-protein diet supplemented by essential amino acids have required SPS continuously, mostly because they were receiving ACE inhibitors; another 20 percent on ACE inhibitors did not develop hyperkalemia. Some patients not on ACE inhibitors nevertheless require SPS. The very-low-protein diet supplemented by essential amino acids may impair potassium excretion because of the decreased amounts of sulfate and phosphate requiring excretion. A fall in the intake of sulfate and phosphate may make hyperkalemia more likely.

The flavored form of amino acids (see Appendix 1) may tend to bind potassium in the gut, acting like SPS.

Potassium Deficiency

Potassium deficiency, manifested as hypokalemia, is much less common. Again, it can be caused by diuretic drugs, such as thiazides, which increase potassium excretion. It can also occur spontaneously. Sometimes the diseased kidneys cannot retain the potassium your body needs.

Occasional patients develop potassium deficiency owing to chronic diarrhea or frequent use of laxatives. In rare cases this can be a primary cause of renal failure.

Unlike hyperkalemia, hypokalemia presents with clear symptoms, including muscle cramps and weakness, which may progress to paralysis. Cardiac rhythm disturbances are often the first manifestation of potassium deficiency, and can be fatal when the potassium deficiency is severe.

Serum potassium concentration below normal, namely less than 3.4 mEq per liter, confirms the diagnosis. Often this also may be associated with an increase in serum bicarbonate concentration, that is, alkalosis.

Treatment of potassium deficiency is simple: oral potassium supplements, such as potassium chloride or potassium bicarbonate. Potassium preparations for oral use are designed so that potassium chloride does not come into contact with the small intestine, where it's known to cause ulcers. The amount of potassium needed to correct and/or prevent deficiency varies; 25 mEq is a good starting dose, but it is usually not enough. Typically the deficiency amounts to 300 mEq or more, so 100 mEq a day would be a good dose. It must be administered slowly to avoid a dangerous rise in serum potassium concentration.

13

Step 9: Treat Calcium and Phosphate Problems

Changes in calcium and phosphate levels in the blood, and consequent disturbances in tissue levels of these minerals, especially in bone, can be major problems for those with severe kidney failure. First, let's review the normal roles of these minerals.

Calcium is the most abundant mineral in the human body, followed by phosphorus. Every plant and animal cell contains some calcium. Calcium combines readily with numerous other elements to form chemical compounds called salts. Calcium salts, such as calcium phosphate in its various forms, are essential not only for the formation of bone, but also for the regulation of many chemical reactions in the body.

Nearly 99 percent of body calcium is stored in the skeleton and about 1 percent in the teeth. But at much lower levels, soluble calcium in body fluids, both inside cells and between cells, plays a critical role in many bodily processes. Calcium ions, which are positively charged, help regulate muscular contractions, including the beating of the heart. They also serve as messengers from the surface of cells to the interior for many physiological functions, such as blood clotting, transmission of nerve impulses, and secretion of hormones.

About one-third of body phosphorus is found in bones in the form of calcium phosphate. Phosphorus is also found in DNA and RNA, the molecules that contain our genetic code. Phosphate bonds are also major storehouses of chemical energy used for muscle contraction and other energy-consuming reactions. Phosphate is also an important component of cell membranes.

In a healthy person, calcium is present at a very constant level in the blood plasma. Phosphate is present at a lower but also a constant level.

Three mechanisms regulate blood calcium concentration:

1. Parathyroid hormone. This hormone is secreted by the parathyroid glands, situated in the neck, in response to a fall in blood calcium concentration. It causes release of calcium from the bones, reduced urinary loss of calcium, and increased production of vitamin D by the kidney.

2. Vitamin D. This vitamin is obtained in part from the diet and is also synthesized in the skin when it is exposed to sunshine. The last step in vitamin D synthesis is carried out in the kidneys and in other tissues, such as the skin. The most important function of vitamin D is to promote the intestinal absorption of calcium, but it has many other functions, some of which have nothing to do with calcium.

3. Calcitonin. This hormone, produced by the thyroid gland, promotes kidney excretion of calcium and inhibits release of calcium from bone. Its effects are the opposite of those of parathyroid hormone.

Blood phosphate concentration is apparently not regulated directly, but rather responds to changes in calcium metabolism. Calcium phosphate is quite insoluble and tends to precipitate out of solution whenever both calcium and phosphate concentration in any solution get high. The product of calcium and phosphate concentration in aqueous solution cannot get above a certain limit. Therefore, when blood phosphate concentration increases, calcium phosphate forms, particularly in soft tissues, lowering both calcium and phosphate levels in the blood. A high intake of phosphate or impairment in the ability of the kidneys to excrete phosphate tends to increase blood phosphate.

What Goes Wrong

In kidney failure, all of these processes are disturbed. Probably the first thing to go is the synthesis of vitamin D by the kidneys, with the result that intestinal absorption of calcium declines. Blood phosphate rises because the kidneys' phosphate excretion is impaired. Both processes tend to lower blood calcium concentration and to stimulate parathyroid hormone secretion. Bone formation is impaired.

Thus, in renal failure, serum phosphate is increased, serum calcium is reduced, serum vitamin D is reduced, parathyroid hormone is increased, and bone biopsy shows changes characteristic of renal failure (renal osteodystrophy). Renal osteodystrophy is a bone disease that is slow to develop and at first produces no symptoms. Sometimes, in fact, patients exhibit no symptoms despite severely abnormal X-rays. But eventually it can be debilitating, especially after dialysis begins. The symptoms include arthritis; bone pain; muscle weakness; spontaneous tendon rupture; itching; abnormalities of the heart, blood vessels, and eyes attributable to calcium phosphate deposits; skeletal deformities; and anemia.

Fortunately, these symptoms can be avoided in patients before dialysis by a supplemented very-low-protein diet that is also low in phosphate, and by oral calcium supplements.

Nevertheless, close examination of patients before dialysis frequently shows early signs of these problems. Patients may have:

- Decreased bone mineral density, most pronounced in the thigh bone (the femur)
- Increased serum levels of parathyroid hormone and phosphorus
- Decreased levels of calcium and vitamin D

Treatment of Calcium and Phosphate Problems

The main features of treatment are to augment calcium intake (as calcium carbonate) and to limit phosphate intake. (See Chapter 7.) About 2 grams of calcium carbonate should be taken daily. Many preparations are available, all equally effective. Phosphate intake should be limited to about 400 mg per day. Blood levels of both parathyroid hormone and vitamin D are more responsive to a low-phosphorus diet than to calcium supplementation.

With such treatment, many of these abnormalities disappear, but sometimes it is necessary to administer an active form of vitamin D. Occasionally it is necessary to surgically remove the parathyroid glands.

In evaluating serum calcium concentration, it is important to recall that about half of serum calcium is bound to albumin. Hence, when albumin concentration is low, total serum calcium may be low even though nonprotein-bound calcium (the biologically important quantity) is normal. A simple formula gives a good estimate of nonprotein-bound calcium (Ca^{2+}) based on total serum calcium (Ca) and albumin (Alb) concentration: $Ca^{2+} = Ca - 1.25(Alb)$. Among my patients, I have rarely seen low levels of nonprotein-bound calcium. High values are even less common.

I have rarely seen excess calcium levels in patients taking calcium carbonate, which is effective even though it is poorly absorbed. Calcium acetate (PhosLo) is better absorbed but may lead to high readings. This may not be a serious problem in dialysis patients, but in predialysis patients, glomerular filtration rate may decrease sharply and may not recover. Calcium carbonate is the much safer option, in my experience.

Serum phosphate in patients on the supplemented very-low-protein diet is usually within normal limits, except in a few patients with very severe renal failure. This is because a low-protein diet is almost always a low-phosphate diet, too; dietary phosphate is highest in foods high in protein. (See chapter 7.)

Some nephrologists have recommended the use of the activated form of vitamin D, calcitriol, in all patients, at a dose of about 0.25 mcg daily. I have used this in a few patients with low serum calcium levels (corrected for albumin) but not otherwise. A recent study from Japan indicates that patients approaching dialysis who have relatively low serum levels of calcitriol are more likely to have low serum levels of albumin, as well. My experience also leads me to believe that the low levels of calcitriol may cause low levels of albumin, but this is an unproven assumption.

If calcitriol treatment is overdone, the first ill effect to be seen is an elevation of serum calcium concentration above normal (hypercalcemia), which can cause a sharp fall in kidney function. Usually kidney function recovers when serum calcium returns to normal, but not always.

As renal failure progresses, phosphate accumulates in the blood, and vitamin D synthesis is further impaired. Both of these changes tend to stimulate the secretion of parathyroid hormone even more. The parathyroid glands enlarge and may in fact get so big that they cannot shut off. As noted earlier, they may have to be surgically removed. These high levels of parathyroid hormone in turn contribute to bone disease, which can be incapacitating in poorly treated patients whose phosphate level stays very high. One sign of this condition is a high level in the blood of the enzyme alkaline phosphatase, released from the bone. Consequent bone pain and fractures can be disabling.

A low-protein, low-phosphate diet, supplemented by ketoacids as calcium salts, may correct this condition completely. Some physicians have maintained that calcium administered as salts of ketoacids is particularly well absorbed. However, this has not been well established, and these salts carry the risk of inducing a high blood calcium concentration.

Alternatively, we can try to reduce intestinal absorption of phosphate. The most commonly used agent for this purpose is calcium carbonate, which, as discussed earlier, should always be part of a low-protein regimen. It combines with phosphate in the gut to form the insoluble salt calcium phosphate, which is excreted in the stool. Many preparations of calcium carbonate are available, generally without a prescription.

In years gone by, patients commonly took aluminum salts, such as aluminum hydroxide, to control phosphate absorption. The body absorbs only small amounts of these salts. Ingestion leads to the formation of another insoluble salt, aluminum phosphate, that is excreted in the stool. These salts are also widely used as antacids. Scientists have established that enough aluminum is absorbed from these salts to cause serious bone damage in patients with chronic renal failure. Nerve and blood cell toxicity also may occur. Today, however, aluminum salts are rarely used to reduce phosphate absorption, and also patients with renal failure should avoid using them as antacids.

Sevelamer, a newly introduced polymer, reduces phosphate absorption and is highly effective but also highly expensive. The more affordable option is for patients to take calcium supplements and reduce phosphate intake.

14

Step 10: Treat Gout and Uric Acid Problems

Gout, called the disease of kings and the king of diseases, has an ancient history. Well known to both the Greeks and the Romans, it is characterized by acute, very painful attacks of arthritis. In 1683 Dr. Thomas Sydenham described a typical first attack in this way:

> The victim goes to bed and sleeps in good health. About two o'clock in the morning, he is awakened by pain in the great toe; more rarely in the heel, ankle or instep. The pain is like that of a dislocation, and yet the parts feel as if cold water were poured over them. Then follows chills and shivers and a little fever. The pain, which was at first moderate, becomes more intense. With its intensity the chills and shivers increase. After a time this comes to its full height. Now it is a violent stretching and tearing of the ligaments—now it is a gnawing pain and now a pressure and tightness. So exquisite and lively meanwhile is the feeling of the part affected, that it cannot bear the weight of bedclothes nor the jar of person walking in the room. The night is passed in torture, sleeplessness, turning of the part affected, and perpetual change of posture.

The duration of an attack of gout varies from a few days to several weeks. When it subsides, the joint returns to its normal state.

The second attack may not occur for one or two years. Subsequently the interval between attacks becomes shorter and shorter, and remission between attacks eventually becomes incomplete; multiple joints become involved, and inflammation may occur in bursae, the small cushions of fluid that facilitate the movement of one structure, such as a tendon, over another.

Gout is a characterized by abnormally high levels of uric acid, a by-product of metabolism, in the blood and tissues. Crystals of uric acid are deposited in the joints, where they cause arthritis. Crystals also may be deposited in the kidneys, where they can lead to kidney damage or to the formation of uric acid kidney stones.

In some patients without kidney disease, high uric acid levels are promoted by a diet rich in purines, which are found in anchovies, nuts, and organ foods such as liver and sweetbreads. More commonly, the body's own production of uric acid is too high, regardless of diet. Factors that increase the likelihood of gout include obesity or sudden weight gain, alcohol intake (especially binge drinking), high blood pressure, family history of gout, trauma or major surgery, and certain types of cancer or cancer treatment. Some 90 percent of patients with gout are over 40 years old, and most are males. Gout is rare in younger women.

Gout and Kidney Failure

Gout is much more frequent in patients with chronic renal failure than in the general population. The explanation lies in the body's control of serum uric acid levels. Uric acid normally is excreted in the urine, but when kidney function decreases, uric acid excretion decreases and, as a result, blood levels tend to rise. An elevation above 6 mg per dl tends to cause precipitation of uric acid in joints (causing gout) and also in the kidneys, sometimes leading to a uric acid kidney stone.

In addition, diuretics such as thiazides and furosemide, which people with kidney disease often use, increase uric acid levels and make gout more likely.

Gout also may be the cause of kidney disease. High uric acid levels (over 13 mg per dl in men and over 10 mg per dl in women) can lead to chronic renal damage.

Treatment

In the absence of kidney disease, the treatment of an acute attack of gout involves the use of a nonsteroidal anti-inflammatory drug (NSAID) (see Chapter 19) or an adrenocortical steroid taken in pill form, or drugs that promote the urinary excretion of uric acid. None of these treatments is safe in people with chronic kidney disease. However, doctors do prescribe allopurinol, which inhibits the production of uric acid whether kidney disease is present or not. Unfortunately, dietary restrictions are of little value in reducing attacks of gout.

When gout occurs in the course of renal failure, patients should avoid NSAIDs, steroids, and drugs that promote uric acid excretion, because all may adversely affect kidney function. Colchicine, a drug that does not injure the kidneys, is available, but it may cause other problems, as detailed below. This drug inhibits the formation of the microcrystals of uric acid that form in joints and give rise to the symptoms of gout. It is given hourly, in doses of 0.65 mg, until diarrhea occurs. By this time the symptoms of gout disappear. In fact, this response is so characteristic that it is used as a diagnostic test for gout. If colchicine does not work, hot soaks of the affected joint may help. In severe cases, it may be necessary to inject cortisol into the affected joint.

Sodium bicarbonate (see Chapter 10) alkalinizes the urine, preventing the formation of uric acid stones, and also may help prevent further kidney damage.

A daily dose of one or two colchicine tablets is also very effective in preventing future attacks, but occasionally such treatment leads to serious or even fatal toxicity. French researchers have described patients with chronic renal failure given 1 mg per day of colchicine (a small dose) who developed severe neuromyopathy (weakness, neuralgia, and muscle dissolution) within a week; two of them died. Clearly, colchicine should *not* be prescribed long term for patients with chronic renal failure.

Patients with elevated serum uric acid concentrations (whether they have kidney disease or not) should be prescribed daily allopurinol, which specifically blocks the synthesis of uric acid. The dose of allopurinol should be sharply reduced in patients with severe renal failure, because their bodies metabolize it more slowly; 50 mg per day or even as little as 25 mg per day may be about right. Some patients show allergic reactions to allopurinol; they may be treated effectively with oxypurinol instead.

Occasional patients exhibit low uric acid levels, reflecting a hereditary defect. This has nothing to do with chronic renal failure, except that such people tend to form kidney stones composed of uric acid and may develop acute kidney failure after exercise. Treatment of uric acid stone-formers is simple: daily doses of sodium bicarbonate. As noted in Chapter 10, this makes uric acid more soluble.

15

Step 11: Treat Your High Cholesterol

In the last 20 years, great strides have been made in increasing public awareness of the dangers of cholesterol. To some degree, we have all become obsessed with the fat and cholesterol content in foods. Manufacturers have taken advantage of our sensitivity, and "fat-free" cookies and cakes and potato chips and "cholesterol-free" eggs and pretzels cram grocery store shelves. But what is cholesterol, and how does it factor into your battle with kidney failure?

What Is Cholesterol?

The truth is we should be concerned with all the fatty substances in the blood serum, known as serum lipids, not just cholesterol. Serum lipids include cholesterol, triglycerides, and little globules of fat known as chylomicrons. These substances play important roles in fat metabolism and also contribute to hardening of the arteries (arteriosclerosis), which is the major cause of coronary heart disease, strokes, and circulatory insufficiency of the legs. This insufficiency causes pain on walking because of inadequate blood flow and can lead to gangrene and the loss of limbs.

Cholesterol is a waxy substance found in all parts of the body. It helps make cell membranes, some hormones, and vitamin D. It comes from two sources: your body and the foods you eat. Cholesterol is made in the liver, and none is necessary in the diet. Dietary cholesterol comes from animal foods such as meats, whole-milk dairy foods, egg yolks, poultry, and fish (especially squid, shrimp, and oysters). Eating too much cholesterol can increase your blood cholesterol level. Foods from plants, such as vegetables, fruits, grains, and cereals, contain no cholesterol.

Two main kinds of fat are found in foods: saturated fats, which contain hydrogen atoms hooked to all of the carbon atoms; and unsaturated fats, which lack some of these hydrogen atoms. High intake of saturated fat, even through no cholesterol is ingested, increases blood cholesterol levels, more than does intake of cholesterol itself, by biochemical mechanisms.

The most widespread defect in American diets (apart from overeating) is high intake of saturated fat, which is responsible for the prevalence of arteriosclerosis. Unsaturated fats, such as olive oil, are much less harmful or may even be beneficial. Therefore, try to cut down on foods high in saturated fats, like fatty meats, cream, and butter, and use olive oil or canola oil.

As is well known, high serum cholesterol levels promote heart disease, and efforts to reduce these levels with diet and drugs are now widespread. Despite this, many Americans are still not sure what cholesterol is, or what they should be doing about it.

In most kidney failure patients, blood cholesterol is no higher than in other people, so their dietary habits with regard to eating cholesterol-containing foods or saturated fats should be the same as in people who don't have kidney disease. There is some evidence that high levels of blood cholesterol increase the rate of loss of kidney function. Thus it becomes even more important for patients with kidney failure to avoid high serum cholesterol levels.

In patients with the nephrotic syndrome (see Chapter 18), cholesterol levels in the blood are typically very high. If this situation is long-standing, it can promote heart disease. But the typical treatment of the nephrotic syndrome does not center on reducing fat intake or the intake of high-cholesterol foods.

The topic of which foods lower serum cholesterol levels and which tend to increase it is very confusing for most people. For example, a product says "no cholesterol" but may contain a lot of saturated fat; consequently, it *increases* serum cholesterol levels. Another product says it is made with vegetable shortening, but the vegetable oil has been hardened by a process called hydrogenation that increases its content of saturated fat.

The two kinds of cholesterol in the blood, "good" cholesterol and "bad" cholesterol, are also very confusing. These terms refer to lipoproteins that carry cholesterol. For reasons only partly understood, the amount of cholesterol bound to one kind of lipoprotein, low-density lipoprotein (LDL), is correlated with the development of arteriosclerosis, while the cholesterol bound to another kind of lipoprotein, high-density lipoprotein (HDL), seems to protect against arteriosclerosis. This is why these two fractions of blood cholesterol sometimes are referred to as "bad" and "good." Most foods that increase cholesterol levels increase LDL cholesterol; HDL cholesterol can be increased by exercise or by moderate amounts of alcohol.

Triglycerides are another fatty substance in the serum that are characteristically elevated in renal failure. The bulk of body fat is in the form of triglycerides, but the serum level in people without kidney failure is usually below 200 mg per dl. There is some evidence that high triglyceride levels in the blood are associated with faster progression of renal insufficiency; it has not been shown yet, however, that lowering the level of triglycerides will slow the progression of kidney failure. The relationship between arteriosclerosis and triglycerides is not as clear cut as the relationship between arteriosclerosis and cholesterol.

Interestingly, high levels of triglycerides and a low level of HDL cholesterol predict the development of kidney disease. Doctors cannot explain this observation, which is based on retrospective analysis of a large number of patients. Patients with renal failure who have high levels of triglycerides should be treated. Fenofibrate is a drug that can safely lower triglyceride levels.

In chronic renal failure, LDL cholesterol is also typically increased (as it is in many people without renal failure). It follows that the supplemented very-low-protein diet, which tends to be somewhat high in fat, should make things worse. Curiously, the opposite seems to be the case: Patients placed on this diet generally exhibit a fall in total and LDL cholesterol and, somewhat less regularly, in triglycerides.

Medications for High Cholesterol

Sometimes, despite making changes to their diet, some people continue to have excessive serum cholesterol concentrations. This situation occurs in patients with the nephrotic syndrome, and in those diabetics who have relatively high rates of protein excretion. These high serum cholesterol levels usually can be treated readily in patients with and without renal failure, including people with diabetes, by the administration of a statin drug. These drugs are just as effective in renal disease as in its absence, and no more toxic. They are being used more and more widely, and seem to have other beneficial effects; some may reduce the incidence of Alzheimer's disease, and some may reduce the incidence of osteoporosis.

If you're taking a statin, your blood should be tested for signs of liver damage at regular intervals; if liver tests become abnormal (at least twice the upper limit of normal), withdrawal of the offending drug and its replacement by another of the same class often is effective, and no clinical liver toxicity results.

Also, muscle damage can occur from statins and can lead to the release into the blood of a protein from damaged muscle, myoglobin, that can cause the kidneys to shut down entirely. This form of acute renal failure has caused the deaths of a number of patients and recently has led to the withdrawal from the market of one of the statins, Baycol. Muscle pain is the first sign of this condition. It also can be detected by monitoring the blood level of an enzyme from muscle called creatine kinase, but this test is not used much for monitoring purposes; muscle pain is more likely to signal this problem.

Despite these dangers, the consensus at present is that statins are worth the risk for people with high levels of cholesterol despite an appropriate diet, and may even be advisable for people whose cholesterol is within normal limits. Clearly people on these drugs should be closely monitored and should be told to quit the drugs if their muscles start to hurt.

16

Step 12: Know the Medications That Slow the Progression of Renal Failure

In this chapter we examine some of the medications that can help your kidney failure from getting any worse. Anyone whose kidney failure is getting worse should receive one of the following drugs, in hopes of slowing down the rate of deterioration, even though the detailed mechanisms by which these drugs work remains to be discovered.

Angiotensin-Converting Enzyme Inhibitors and Angiotensin Receptor Blockers

Both angiotensin-converting enzyme inhibitors (ACEIs) and angiotensin receptor blockers (ARBs) reduce angiotensin action. Angiotensin, a powerful hormone, has many actions, the most important of which is constriction of small blood vessels, leading to a rise in blood pressure and therefore in the pressure of blood within the glomerular capillaries in the kidneys. Lowering this pressure may well be the mechanism by which these drugs tend to slow progression of kidney failure.

The effects of ACEIs differ from those of ARBs in several important respects. It is even conceivable that taking drugs from both classes is more effective than taking just one or the other alone. Unfortunately, side-to-side comparisons of these two classes of drugs have not been performed, because the drug industry has no interest in such trials. These drugs are also effective in reducing urinary protein excretion in the nephrotic syndrome, and they also slow progression of chronic renal failure even when added to a low-protein diet.

Many clinical trials have demonstrated slowed progression with ACEIs, and more recently with ARBs, particularly in patients who have large amounts of urinary protein. Yet surprisingly, some recent evidence has indicated that ACEIs are no more effective than calcium channel blockers (see Chapter 9) in slowing the progression of diabetic kidney disease. Whether ACEIs and ARBs have unusual "renoprotective" effects remains unsettled. The bulk of evidence indicates that they do. However, with prolonged administration, urinary protein loss resumes in nearly half the patients, and they subsequently develop worsening kidney function.

An increasing number of patients, particularly older men, exhibit a sharp deterioration of kidney function when placed on ACEIs or ARBs. The majority of patients with severe renal failure exhibit a smaller drop in glomerular filtration rate (GFR; usually manifested as a rise in creatinine concentration) when they are placed on these drugs. This drop presages subsequent slower progression. In other words, the more that GFR falls initially, the less it will fall subsequently. Patients who are dehydrated, as a result of diuretic treatment or gastrointestinal fluid loss, and patients who have heart failure and are taking these drugs, are particularly susceptible to a drop in GFR and may have a severe decrease in renal function.

Cough is a common side effect of ACEIs (though not of ARBs). Frequently, the cause is not identified, and doctors may prescribe extensive testing for pulmonary or laryngeal disease. Once the drug is withdrawn, the cough subsides in a few weeks.

Chapter 12 considers the problem of high blood potassium with these classes of drugs.

Ketoconazole and Low-Dose Prednisone

Ketoconazole (Nizoral) has been used extensively to treat fungal infections for a number of years. Ketoconazole also is used in renal transplant recipients to reduce the rate of metabolism of cyclosporine, thereby lowering the dosage requirement of this expensive drug.

Ketoconazole inhibits the synthesis of cortisol, the main glucocorticoid hormone produced by the adrenal cortex. High rates of production of cortisol are associated with faster progression of chronic renal failure, while low rates of cortisol production are associated with slow progression or no progression.

These observations led us to the hypothesis that ketoconazole administration on a long-term basis might slow the progression of renal failure. One problem with this concept is the well-known "escape" phenomenon: When cortisol production is inhibited, adrenocorticotrophic hormone (ACTH), derived from the pituitary gland, increases and stimulates the adrenal gland to produce more cortisol. We have found that this "escape" can be prevented by administering a low dose (2.5 mg per day) of prednisone (a synthetic glucocorticoid) at the same time. ACTH levels do not rise, and the block in cortisol synthesis persists.

Ketoconazole has other effects that might lead to slower progression of renal disease.

We have published the results of our study on the effect of ketoconazole (200 mg per day) plus low-dose prednisone (2.5 mg per day) in 27 patients with chronic renal failure. In diabetic nephropathy, glomerular diseases, and interstitial nephritis, we observed distinct slowing of progression. In polycystic kidney disease, however, progression was not slowed and may have been accelerated. A discussion of long-term results of taking ketoconazole plus low-dose prednisone in two patients with diabetic kidney disease follows.

Eve Magee, a 47-year-old black curriculum specialist in the Baltimore City school system, was referred in April 1998. She had been diabetic for 19 years, and had been on insulin for several years. Kidney involvement was first detected one year earlier, but high blood pressure had been present for two years, treated with a variety of drugs. Serum creatinine most recently was reported as 4.7 mg per dl, and urine protein as 1.9 g per day. For seven months she had been getting injections of erythropoietin. She was free of symptoms, except for some numbness and tingling in her feet. Her mother and a sister were diabetic, too. Physical exam was negative except for systolic hypertension (blood pressure 170/65) and ankle swelling. Laboratory reports came back as follows: serum creatinine 3.9 mg per dl, serum urea nitrogen 69 mg per dl, urine protein 2.53 g per day, glomerular filtration rate 11 ml per min. She was instructed on a very-low-protein diet (0.3 g per kg) and told how to get essential amino acids. Three weeks later serum urea nitrogen had fallen to normal (23 mg per dl). At this point she was started on ketoconazole and low-dose prednisone. We did not measure her rate of loss of kidney function first during a control period, because of the severity of her renal failure. She took 200 mg per day of keto-conazole and 2.5 mg per day of prednisone daily for the next four years. The only problem that arose was that the transplant service had worked her up for a transplant and called to tell her that a kidney had become available. Since she had no symptoms and was not progressing, she declined. However, she recently developed pneumonia, and never regained her vigor afterward. She finally went on dialysis, having deferred it for about four years.

—Dialysis deferral: 4 years

Larry Phee, a former government employee ("paper shuffler," in his words), came to Johns Hopkins eight years ago at age 67, with a 40-year history of insulin-dependent diabetes.

For five years he had known of kidney involvement, and also had been hypertensive. Urinary protein was said to be 0.8 to 1.0 g per day, but we found only about 350 mg per day. He had been on insulin, an ACE inhibitor, and allopurinol. He had restricted dietary protein to about 50 g per day. His symptoms included muscle cramps, impotence, loss of vision, and neuralgia. Nevertheless, he got regular exercise and kept his blood sugar very well controlled. There was a strong family history of diabetes. Except for diabetic retinal damage, his physical exam was normal. He was not started on a very-low-protein diet initially, because his symptoms didn't warrant it. Throughout 1994 and 1995, his

GFR fell progressively, and in 1995 he was started on a very-low-protein diet supplemented by essential amino acids, despite the absence of symptoms. Progression continued. In 1996, 200 mg per day of keto-conazole, and 2.5 mg per day of prednisone were added. At that time his GFR was 33.8 ml per min. Seven years later, it is only slightly lower (29.5 ml per min on July 18, 2003). Thus progression of his kidney disease has stopped. Between July 1999 and June 2000, he had problems with high blood potassium, owing to the ACE inhibitor and the reluctance of his primary physician to discontinue it. When it was finally discontinued (June 2000), urinary protein excretion initially increased but has now fallen again to 384 mg per day. He has no symptoms of renal failure and swims every day for 40 minutes.

—Dialysis deferral: 7 years so far

One problem with ketoconazole is the occurrence of early signs of liver damage in a substantial proportion of patients. We stopped the drug in 20 percent of our patents when abnormal blood tests warned of impending liver damage (or because of other side effects). The blood tests soon returned to normal, and no clinically significant liver damage occurred. But it is important to note that continuance of ketoconazole despite abnormal liver function tests may lead to severe and even fatal liver disease.

The chances of an individual developing clinically significant liver toxicity in a year of treatment with ketoconazole are 1.6 percent, based on international experience with this drug. Careful monitoring of serum enzyme levels should prevent significant liver toxicity altogether, as it has in our small series.

Ketoconazole also has a number of lesser side effects that often disappear with continued administration. These include fatigue, headache, light sensitivity, and others. Apparently the side effects and adverse effects of ketoconazole are no different in people with kidney disease from the effects seen in people without kidney disease.

At this low dosage, prednisone has no side effects.

Unfortunately, because the patent on ketoconazole has expired, further studies of its use to slow the progression of kidney failure will not be performed, unless the government takes an interest. The drug industry has no interest in doing studies of drugs with expired patents. Nevertheless, your doctor can prescribe ketoconazole and prednisone for you. The Food and Drug Administration permits physicians to prescribe drugs for "off-label" uses, meaning uses that have not been established to be safe and effective in large drug trials and hence have not been officially approved. When physicians do prescribe drugs for off-label uses, they have to monitor the patients carefully. In the case of ketoconazole, this means keeping a close eye on liver tests.

PART III

TRACKING KIDNEY FAILURE, DIALYSIS OPTIONS, TRANSPLANTS, AND MORE

This section includes information that will aid you in keeping track of your kidney failure (whether you have slowed the progression of your disease, or whether your renal failure is still getting worse), and what to do if you have to go on dialysis, as well as consider kidney transplantation. There is also information in this section for those suffering from the nephrotic syndrome.

17

Keeping Close Watch on Your Kidney Failure

This chapter is an important one to read to find out more about how your kidney failure is diagnosed and measured, whether your disease is being measured accurately, and whether you are getting worse. You do not need to read this chapter to find out the best way to treat your kidney failure effectively. But if you like to be well informed about the details of your disease, please read on. The information provided is particularly useful for people with kidney failure because, as noted earlier, physical symptoms are not a reliable guide to judging the severity of kidney failure or to the rate at which kidney function is decreasing. Lab measurements are the key.

Diagnosing and Measuring Kidney Failure

How can kidney failure be diagnosed?

Kidney disease can be detected by imaging techniques, such as X rays of the abdomen, sonograms of the kidneys, or intravenous pyelograms. But with the exception of X rays, which might show small kidneys (indicating the presence of renal failure), imaging techniques are ordered only if kidney disease is already suspected. Thus these techniques are not generally a means of detecting kidney disease, even though they can be definitive if kidney failure is already suspected. The best screening test for chronic renal impairment is on a sample of blood. Let's find out why blood constituents change in concentration in early kidney failure.

Urine contains hundreds of known constituents. A few of these are produced in the kidney, but the vast majority are derived from the blood. Day after day, each of these constituents is being added to the bloodstream continuously, either derived from the diet or produced by the metabolic activity of one organ or another, and is then removed by the kidney at the same rate (on average). Thus the concentration in the blood of each constituent fluctuates around some average value. Long term, the rate at which each of these urinary constituents appears in the bloodstream is the same as the rate at which it is being excreted. So even if there are short-term fluctuations in the level in the blood, the average concentration, over time, tends to be constant.

Consider now what would happen if one kidney were removed. The remaining kidney would excrete any given constituent at a rate half as great as did two kidneys before. The constituent would therefore accumulate in the body, causing a progressive rise in its concentration in the blood and in its rate of excretion. Eventually, a new steady state would be reached, such that the rate of production of the substance by the body (or rate of its addition to the body by the diet) would again be equal to its rate of excretion, at least on a daily basis. We would find that its concentration in the blood is twice normal, and we therefore could infer that kidney function was one-half of normal. If its measured concentration in the blood were four times normal, we would infer that kidney function was one-quarter of normal. If the measured concentration were five times normal, we could infer that kidney function was one-fifth of normal, and so forth.

This reciprocal relationship is very useful in the evaluation of kidney disease. Measurement of some such constituent in the blood is essential to assessing how well the kidneys are working. Unfortunately, no ideal substance for this purpose has been identified yet, and all such measurements are subject to some error.

For the results to come out as predicted by the reciprocal relationship described earlier, two conditions must be met:

1. The rate at which the constituent is entering the bloodstream

(from diet or from metabolism) would have to be constant from day to day, and fluctuations in its production rate would have to be minor.

2. Exact proportionality would have to exist between the concentration of the constituent in the blood and its rate of excretion by the kidney. More precisely, the ratio of the excretion to blood concentration (known as clearance) would have to be a constant at any level of kidney function.

No known constituent meets these requirements. However, a few come close.

The substances that come closest are not naturally occurring constituents but they can be injected. Obviously they also must be nontoxic. It is hoped that their only fate in the body is removal by the kidney; that is, no other organ metabolizes them to any significant extent. (This last condition turns out to be the hardest to meet.)

Inulin, a sugar polymer obtained from the Jerusalem artichoke, was the first such substance identified. The earliest quantitative studies of kidney function, 75 years ago, were made with the aid of inulin. Several other substances subsequently have been identified that meet the required conditions for this use, some radioactive and some nonradioactive. They are known as glomerular filtration markers. These other substances are usually employed in place of inulin, because inulin is difficult to obtain, difficult to work with, and difficult to measure. When one of these glomerular filtration markers is infused intravenously at a constant rate, its concentration in the blood and its rate of excretion in the urine gradually increase until a steady state is reached. At that point the rate of filtration by the glomeruli and rate of excretion in the urine are exactly equal to the marker's rate of infusion. The more glomeruli are operative, the lower the final concentration. If total kidney function is halved, the final concentration in the blood is doubled, and so forth.

The time required for the final concentration to be achieved depends on the amount of kidney function. In a healthy person, it takes several hours; in someone with severe kidney failure, it may take as long as two days. Because the marker substance must be infused continuously throughout this time, the patient must wear a constant infusion pump on a belt, attached to an intravenous line.

How can we use the known rate of infusion of this substance and its final steady-state concentration to determine the rate of glomerular filtration? Since the concentration of the marker in the filtrate is the same as its concentration in blood plasma, the amount of filtrate formed per unit of time, in ml per minute, is simply the excretion rate (or infusion rate) of the marker divided by this final concentration. This quotient is the volume of fluid having a concentration the same as this final plasma concentration. This volume of fluid is being formed in each unit of time. Called the glomerular filtration rate (GFR), it is the only good measure of the amount of kidney function remaining.

Normally GFR is about 100 ml per minute. In kidney failure, GFR decreases progressively; when it gets below 5 to 10 ml per minute, dialysis or transplantation is necessary for survival.

We have also described the principle of renal clearance: The rate of excretion of any substance divided by its plasma concentration is its plasma clearance. The clearance of glomerular filtration markers is the glomerular filtration rate. If a substance is also added to the tubular fluid by tubular secretion, its clearance will be greater than the GFR. If a substance is partially reabsorbed by the tubules, its clearance will be less than the GFR. Some of the substances recommended for measuring various aspects of kidney function have clearances that are greater or less than the GFR.

Finding Your Glomerular Filtration Rate

There are four distinct ways of measuring GFR:

1. The constant infusion technique
2. Via intravenous injections
3. Via urine samples
4. Via radioactive markers

The Constant Infusion Technique

In the constant infusion technique, a marker substance is infused continuously into a vein at a constant rate by means of a pump (which may be a portable device strapped around the waist), until the plasma concentration becomes constant. The known infusion rate is divided by this final concentration to obtain GFR in ml per minute. There is no need to collect urine. Curiously, this technique, although known for decades, has been employed in the evaluation of chronic renal failure only in the last few years. It is particularly useful in children, in whom it is more difficult to obtain timed samples of urine, but a good case can be made that it also should be used in adults. There are four disadvantages:

1. The marker substance must not be removed by any other organ, as noted earlier.

2. When kidney function is severely impaired, the steady state is reached only after a day or two of infusion, which is inconvenient to say the least.

3. Reliable portable constant infusion pumps are quite expensive.

4. The ideal marker substance to use in this technique is still being sought.

Nevertheless, wider use of this technique is likely to develop because of its accuracy and simplicity.

Intravenous Injections

In a modification of the constant infusion technique that is very widely used, a GFR substance is injected intravenously, and its disappearance from the body is measured by several blood samples obtained during the ensuing hours. Many different formulas have been proposed for calculating GFR from timed blood samples. No urine samples are required, but this technique suffers from the same disadvantage as the constant infusion technique, namely, that removal of the marker by organs other than the kidney causes errors, which become amplified as the removal rate by the kidney decreases (in severe renal failure).

Urine Samples

The urinary clearance method, the conventional method for measuring GFR, involves collecting and analyzing timed urine samples (usually three) while the marker is infused intravenously at a constant rate. Blood samples also are obtained during each collection period. The rate of excretion of the marker during each collection period is divided by the average plasma concentration during the period, to obtain its clearance, which is equal to the GFR during that period. The three estimates of GFR are then averaged.

The urinary clearance technique cannot be used if complete urine collections cannot be obtained. Many persons do not empty their bladders completely when they void, for a variety of reasons. For example, people with diabetes may have some degenerative changes in the nerves that supply the bladder. Older men often have some degree of prostate enlargement that causes residual urine to remain in the bladder after voiding. Patients whose kidney failure is the late result of congenital defects in the urinary system, many of whom develop enlarged bladders, often continue to have substantial residual urine in the bladder after voiding.

The greater the rate of urine flow, the more likely is complete emptying of the bladder. Consequently, someone undergoing this test will be encouraged to take steps to increase urine flow during the measurement of GFR. Drinking four glasses of water about an hour before the procedure starts usually will increase urine flow substantially. During the procedure, it is only necessary to continue to drink an amount of water roughly equal in volume to the volume of urine voided. In this way, the body maintains a constant water load. The water loading is begun an hour before the test because it takes an hour or so for antidiuretic hormone to disappear, after a drop in the concentration of dissolved solutes in body fluids signals the need to do so.

It is important to note that water loading can be overdone, with serious consequences. Many patients believe that the more water they drink, the better their GFR result will be. As far as I know, it is not possible to increase GFR at all by water loading; in fact, water loading may decrease GFR. However, a high urine flow does make it easier to measure.

Too much water loading can lead to a severe headache, nausea, vomiting, and even convulsions. This problem tends to be self-perpetuating, because nausea and pain are powerful stimuli for the secretion of antidiuretic hormone. Thus the patient's discomfort, brought on by too much water loading and/or by painful attempts to draw blood, may in itself make it difficult to urinate. Eventually, though, the water load is excreted and all symptoms disappear.

The major problem with the urinary clearance technique, as I noted earlier, is errors caused by incomplete urine collections. Detecting these errors is problematic in itself. Some physicians discard any results based on an arbitrary lower limit of urine flow rate, say 1 ml per minute. Another technique can be employed only if the marker substance is a gamma ray–emitting radioactive tracer. It involves determining the fraction of each voiding that remains in the bladder by measuring the radioactive emissions over the bladder before and after voiding. Using an ultrasound device to determine the amount of residual urine after voiding is another option.

It is hoped that one of these techniques will reduce the errors caused by incomplete voiding. These errors become more problematic as renal failure becomes more severe, because the maximal urine flow (during water loading) falls along with the fall in GFR. Nevertheless, we have been able to obtain consistent GFR results in patients with GFRs as low as 3 or 4 ml per minute, in whom urine flow during the test does not exceed 1 ml per minute. Many patients achieve better urine flow if they remain recumbent during the procedure.

Radioactive Markers

A fourth technique involves measuring radioactivity over the kidney after injecting the patient with a gamma ray–emitting radioactive marker. So far, at least, this technique gives results that correspond very poorly to results obtained by some of the techniques already mentioned, especially in patients with chronic renal failure.

Normal Values for GFR

What is a normal GFR? Normal values are usually expressed as a function of body surface area (BSA), even though this is less than an ideal referent. Bigger people have higher GFRs. Body surface area is obtained from height and weight. An average size man or woman (BSA = 1.73 m^2) would be expected to have a GFR of about 100 ml per min.

The Blood Analysis Method for Assessing Kidney Function Using Naturally Occurring Substances

All of these techniques for measuring GFR, like the imaging techniques mentioned earlier, are unsatisfactory as screening methods, because they are too expensive and too invasive.

We therefore return to the question of whether a substance produced in the body comes reasonably close to meeting the conditions set forth earlier. There are three candidates: creatinine, urea, and cystatin C.

Creatinine

Creatinine is produced continuously in the body by the spontaneous breakdown of creatine (a constituent of muscle) to creatinine. It is scarcely broken down at all in the body (at least in normal subjects) and is excreted unchanged in the urine. An increase in plasma or serum creatinine concentration is undoubtedly the most commonly used screening test for early kidney impairment. Furthermore, a doubling of serum creatinine concentration does indicate that renal function is reduced by approximately half; a five-fold increase indicates that renal function is reduced to approximately one-fifth; and so forth—similar to the idealized relationship described earlier. Normal serum creatinine concentrations are less than 1.5 mg per ml (in men) or 1.4 mg per ml (in women).

Despite its simplicity, there are major disadvantages to using creatinine level as a measure of kidney function.

First, creatinine is derived not only from the spontaneous breakdown of muscle creatine but also from the diet. For example, meat contains creatine, and if the meat you eat is well cooked, some or all of this creatine will be converted to creatinine and will be excreted in the urine. Intact creatine in food goes into muscle, increasing the store of creatine in muscle, and other tissues, leading eventually to an increase in the rate of production of creatinine. About 15 percent of urinary creatinine is derived from the diet in these two ways, but the proportion varies enormously. Patients with chronic renal failure are often on low-protein diets, so that in these people in particular, creatinine derived from the diet may be exceptionally low.

Second, variations between individuals in the amount of muscle mass will cause parallel variations in the amount of creatinine produced by breakdown of creatine in muscle. A given degree of elevation of serum creatinine in an old woman indicates much more severe impairment of kidney function than the same degree of elevation in a muscular young man.

Third, and most important, creatinine is not only filtered by the glomeruli; the renal tubules also secrete it into the urine. The extent of this secretion varies enormously from one subject to another and also from day to day in a given subject. As a result, the urinary clearance of creatinine exceeds the GFR by a variable amount that may be as much as twofold, or as little as zero. Thus, creatinine clearance is a very poor measure of kidney function. Many authors have recommended that the measurement of 24-hour creatinine clearance be abandoned, but most hospitals still offer this test.

Creatinine does not meet the proportionality between reciprocal concentration and kidney function.

Cimetidine-Modified Creatinine Clearance

About 10 years ago, several researchers reported that cimetidine, a widely used drug for the treatment of an overly acidic stomach, blocks the tubular secretion of creatinine. It was suggested that urinary creatinine clearance measured after cimetidine administration might be a reliable index of GFR. More than a dozen studies have now been published comparing GFR measured by the constant infusion of a GFR marker substance with the simultaneous clearance of creatinine after administering cimetidine. In general, the correspondence is quite close. Our own results, using doses of 900 mg cimetidine the night before the study and again the morning of the study, confirm this. In 31 of 32 patients, creatinine clearance measured in this manner was only slightly (average 7 percent) greater than GFR.

In the thirty-second subject, the discrepancy was much greater, even on repeated measurements. We never could explain this aberrant result, but he is the only one of more than 250 patients in the literature, studied with simultaneous measurements of radioisotopes and creatinine after cimetidine, in whom such a large discrepancy has been observed. Perhaps one of the many drugs he was taking was responsible for the discrepancy.

In the remaining subjects, the rate of progression of renal failure, estimated from sequential measurements of GFR, did not differ (on the average) from the rate of progression measured from sequential creatinine clearances. We conclude that this technique of measuring GFR is a practical and reliable alternative that gives results very close to GFR measurements in most subjects. We have observed no side effects from cimetidine in these patients; only one of the many other articles on this technique has reported any side effects, which were not severe.

It is hoped that this technique will be used more and more.

The Cimetidine-Modified Creatinine Clearance Technique

Most clinics are not set up to collect timed urine samples from patients (although they formerly did this frequently). You can collect the samples yourself. First you need to get your doctor to give you signed lab requisitions for creatinine on three urine samples and one blood sample. Then you need to get cimetidine (available without a prescription) from your pharmacy. Tablets of 300 mg tablets may be available, in which case you need to take three tablets the night before the test and three more the morning of the test. If 300 mg tablets are not available, take four 200 mg tablets instead, both the night before the test and the morning of the test. You also need to buy a 250 ml graduated cylinder (preferably plastic) to measure your urine volume. The morning of the test, take your medications as usual but eat either a light breakfast or no breakfast (because a large meal changes kidney function). Slowly drink four glasses of water or clear beverage. After an hour or so, void and note the time exactly. Then collect three consecutive 30- to 40-minute urine samples, carefully noting the time and total volume of each. If your urine flow seems too low, trying lying down. If you void large volumes, drink some more water. Get the lab to draw one blood sample during the test. Send the blood sample and portions of the three urine samples to the lab with the requisitions. It will send the results of the creatinine measurements to your doctor, who can calculate your creatinine clearance from these data or can show you how to do it (it's very simple). This is your glomerular filtration rate.

When collection of timed urine samples is not possible, it is common practice to estimate GFR from serum creatinine alone. Formulas have been proposed for estimating GFR from serum creatinine concentration, weight, age, and gender. This approach is very unreliable, for reasons already given. It can yield misleading estimates of the rate of progression: Progression may be thought to be occurring when it is not, or vice versa. Presumably this is because the rate of tubular secretion of creatinine varies considerably over time in a given individual.

Specifically, GFR, in ml per min is very roughly given by the formula $(86/[Cr]) - 4.3$ in men and $(69/[Cr]) - 3.8$ in women, where $[Cr]$ is the serum creatinine concentration in mg per dl. These equations are not valid if $[Cr]$ is less than 2 mg per dl. They are included here just for the sake of completenesss. Better equations take into account age and weight, but the errors are enormous. There are much better alternatives for assessing kidney function (see below).

A good case can be made that creatinine, measured in blood (or in 24-hour urine samples as well as blood) without cimetidine pretreatment, should be abandoned. A better alternative is creatinine measured after cimetidine pretreatment, or, better yet, cystatin C level in the blood (see below). But change in medicine is slow, and doctors are not about to stop evaluating kidney function from creatinine measurements without cimetidine pretreatment.

To get some idea of what various levels of serum creatinine concentration mean, the average concentration at which patients go on to dialysis is about 8 mg per dl, although some begin at levels as low as 3 mg per dl. The highest creatinine concentration I have ever heard of was 46 mg per dl in a man who walked into the emergency room with no complaints related to renal failure. When creatinine concentration is between 1.5 mg per dl (the upper limit of the normal range) and 2 mg per dl, other equations have been proposed, but they are very rough approximations. In half of patients with 40 to 80 percent of kidney function left, creatinine concentration is still normal, that is, less than 1.5 mg per dl.

When plugged into a formula that takes age, gender, and weight into consideration, cimetidine pretreatment may not only give a good estimate of GFR from serum creatinine concentration alone without urine measurement, but also may be a reliable way to follow the progression of kidney failure. Apparently there are no side effects of cimetidine to worry about when given in this way.

Urea

Another candidate substance for a naturally occurring marker of kidney function is urea. Like creatinine, urea is produced continuously in the body, being the principal end product of protein metabolism, and is excreted in the urine. As you would expect, its rate of production is highly dependent on protein intake. Severe protein restriction can reduce urea production so much that its concentration in the blood can be close to normal even in severe renal failure. At the opposite extreme, very high levels of protein intake can increase blood urea concentration so much that renal failure is falsely diagnosed.

This was illustrated by the following case, reported in *The Lancet* in 1975.

A 49-year-old woman related that she had had a poor appetite since age 19. She had learned that she could remain thin by eating large quantities of protein, specifically codfish, which she consumed in enormous quantities (up to 3 pounds a day). She also took a milk protein powder, small amounts of cauliflower, cabbage, and cottage cheese, and drank only black coffee. Her protein intake was estimated to average about 400 g per day. Despite normal kidney function, her blood urea nitrogen concentration was repeatedly found to be very high—about 70 mg per dl (the upper limit of normal is 22 mg per dl).

From this example, we might assume that urea concentration is worthless as an index of kidney function. In fact, it is very useful, because most people consume about the same amount of protein daily, 50 to 100 grams. Extreme examples like the case just cited are uncommon. Another reason is that the symptoms and signs of kidney failure, described in the following chapter, are related in severity to the degree of elevation of blood urea concentration (among other abnormalities). This is not because urea itself is toxic (although it does become toxic at very high levels), but rather because urea accumulation reflects the accumulation of many other products of protein metabolism, many of which probably are more toxic than urea.

Urea clearance is always, or nearly always, less than GFR, because the kidney tubules partially reabsorb urea. The ratio of urea clearance to GFR is extremely variable in normal persons, but tends to become more nearly constant as kidney failure becomes more severe.

Normal urea nitrogen concentration = 6 to 22 mg per 100 ml
Abnormal urea nitrogen concentration = greater than 22 mg per 100 ml

Thus urea concentration is a useful marker for kidney failure, but it must be interpreted in the light of known protein intake.

There are several other constituents of the blood whose level of accumulation, in patients with chronic kidney disease, reflects the severity of renal failure. None of these substances, however, is widely used to determine the level of kidney function, although several have been advocated for that purpose.

Cystatin C

Cystatin C, a low-molecular-weight protein that circulates in the blood, appears to be a promising candidate; in fact, in every way it appears to be better than creatinine to determine the level of kidney function. It is not secreted by kidney tubules, so it is not necessary to administer a drug to inhibit tubular secretion before measuring it. Measurement of cystatin C is more reliable than creatinine in early renal failure. It is also more reliable in people with liver disease, in whom creatinine levels become particularly unreliable. Further studies may result in cystatin C taking the place of creatinine as the standard marker for kidney function.

Everyone with chronic kidney disease should have GFR measured periodically by one of the methods just described. There is simply no other good way to assess severity or rate of progression of the disease. The cimetidine-modified creatinine clearance technique has made periodic testing practical.

For some reason, few institutions offer GFR measurement as a diagnostic test, and few physicians request it. No one hesitates to measure changes in visual acuity (in patients who are losing their vision) or audiograms (in patients who are losing their hearing), but hardly anyone measures sequential changes in GFR in patients whose kidneys are failing. One reason may be the exorbitant prices that some hospitals charge for GFRs. Another reason is the widespread skepticism about the utility of predialysis treatment. Documentation, by sequential GFRs, of the progressive loss of kidney function is not a justifiable healthcare expense if, as some believe, nothing can be done to alter this process.

The thesis of this book, however, is that the opposite is the case: Loss of kidney function can be slowed. It follows that regular measurements of kidney function, using the most precise techniques available, are not only eminently worthwhile, but are a requirement of good care. Perhaps someday a self-test for serum creatinine or serum cystatin will become available, like self-tests for blood glucose that are widely used by people with diabetes.

The 24-Hour Urine Test

Another worthwhile lab test for people with kidney disease is the measurement of protein and urea nitrogen in a 24-hour urine collection. Measurement in a single urine sample is less informative, because it varies considerably from hour to hour. A 24-hour urine collection gives a much more precise estimate of just how much protein the kidneys are spilling and how much urea is being produced.

The 24-hour urea nitrogen excretion test is the best measure of how much protein you are eating, because almost all protein eaten is metabolized to urea. Various reports have appeared in which the reliability of "spot" urine samples is compared with 24-hour collections: Clearly the latter are preferable, even though they are much more trouble for the patient.

The technique of collecting the 24-hour sample is this: On awakening, the patient voids in the toilet as usual. From then on, all urine passed goes into a container, which is kept in the refrigerator, including the urine passed on awakening the following morning. It is important to remember to void in the container before having a bowel movement, because otherwise some urine may be lost. The completed collection can be kept in the refrigerator several days if necessary, but most patients collect it the day before their appointment with the doctor. If any urine is lost, you must start over; an incomplete collection is worse than none at all.

One problem that sometimes arises is finding a large enough container. Using more than one container for the 24-hour collection is problematic, because the lab must find a single large container to mix it all together, and sometimes it cannot to do this. Gallon plastic jugs are easy to come by, as milk and spring water are sold this way. A good rinsing with hot water is adequate. But some patients pass more than a gallon of urine a day as a result of problems with their kidneys' ability to conserve water. How does one locate a two-gallon container? The only answer I can give is to go and buy a big container of kitty litter, dump it out, and rinse it thoroughly. These plastic jugs can hold several gallons and have a handle.

From the 24-hour urea nitrogen excretion level, your doctor can calculate just how much protein you are eating, which will tell you how well you are following the diet.

Tracking Treatment Success

Many treatments have been advocated to slow the downhill course of kidney failure. Before one can evaluate the effect of any treatment, though, a good method for measuring the rate of loss of kidney function is necessary. Traditionally creatinine levels have been used for this purpose. When these values are plotted as reciprocals against time, they usually form a straight line. (See Figure 17.1A and Figure 17.1B.) If creatinine values are plotted against time without taking reciprocals first, you may get the impression that the progress of your kidney failure is accelerating, when it is in fact progressing at a constant rate. The reason for this result is: If creatinine excretion (UV) remains constant and kidney function (creatinine clearance, UV/P) steadily declines, then 1/P must decline steadily too (Figure 17.1B). The slope of this line is a measure of progression (it needs to be multiplied by an average value of 24-hour creatinine excretion, UV, in mg per day, in order to come out in units of GFR change, in ml per min per mo).

FIGURE 17.1A AND 17.1B

Time course of an "ideal filtration marker" (see text) as kidney function declines in a patient with kidney disease.

Assumption 1: Kidney function, calculated as the rate of excretion of the marker divided by its plasma concentration, P, declines steadily with time.

Assumption 2: Excretion of the marker, which is produced by the body at the constant rate, remains constant with time, despite decreasing kidney function.

Consequence 1: Plasma concentration, P, of the marker increases at a progressively increasing rate with time, even though kidney function is declining at a steady rate (Figure 17.1A).

Consequence 2: The reciprocal of plasma concentration, 1/P, declines at a constant rate with time (Figure 17.1B). This rate is a measure of how fast kidney function is decreasing.

FIGURE 17.1A

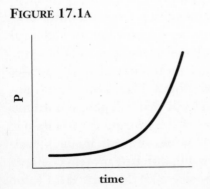

FIGURE 17.1B

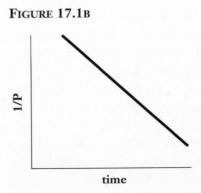

This technique, even though it is widely used, is very unreliable. Thus, based on sequential creatinine measurements, progression may appear from to be occurring when in fact it is not, and the converse is also true. These problems occur whether the measurements consist of creatinine levels alone or of creatinine clearances (without cimetidine). Furthermore, not all patients' creatinine measurements yield a straight line when plotted.

As summarized earlier, cimetidine, administered the night before a clearance test and again at the start of the determination, makes creatinine clearance nearly equal to GFR (actually about 7 percent greater), when measured over three 30- to 40-minute collection periods, with water loading. Furthermore, the rate of progression, measured by sequential values of creatinine clearance (or, more simply, serum creatinine values, recalculated as reciprocals, after taking cimetidine each time), is equal to the rate of progression measured simultaneously in the same subjects by radioactive isotope GFR determinations. This technique is a relatively simple and inexpensive way to assess disease progression.

It is paradoxical that serum creatinine concentration, the most widely employed measure of kidney function, should be so highly unreliable by itself, but it should become so reliable after cimetidine administration.

A modification of simply measuring sequential creatinine concentrations has been used in clinical trials: The time to doubling of serum creatinine concentration of each patient is calculated, and the results for each treatment group are averaged and compared. A major difficulty with this technique is that in some patients, serum creatinine concentrations fail to double in the allotted interval. This will be the case no matter how long the interval, because, as explained in Chapter 16, for unknown reasons, some patients never do progress. This technique has little to recommend it.

Until recently it was generally agreed that only sequential measurements of GFR could give reliable estimates of progression for a clinical trial. Even with these measurements, problems arose. For example, it is well recognized that GFR, in the presence or absence of renal disease, varies with protein intake. Thus a normal subject, placed on a very-low-protein diet, will experience a decrease in GFR that will persist until the subject goes off the diet. The magnitude of this change is variable but averages about 20 percent; it takes several weeks to reach its final level. Any study comparing progression on diets with differing protein contents must deal with this short-term effect. In particular, if the starting GFR for each patient is taken as the baseline GFR, before starting a low-protein diet, the actual rate of progression on the low-protein diet will be over-estimated, sometimes by a considerable amount. What matters to the patient's future is the long-term rate of progression, not the degree of decline in a relatively short period. A French study of disease progression on people taking ketoacids failed to find an effect because the researchers did not consider this problem. This phenomenon also has obscured the con-clusions of the large Modification of Diet in Renal Disease Study, in which those on protein restriction clearly exhibited a short-term decline in GFR and a later reduced rate of progression. When the study ended at two years, there was little difference between final GFRs of the two groups, even though the disease clearly was progressing more slowly among those whose protein intake was lower.

So far we have assumed that GFR measurements are to be taken at regular intervals, and the rate of decline of GFR calculated from these data. It turns out that this approach is quite inefficient. The GFR meas-urements at the beginning and end of the period of observation have a much more important effect in determining the rate of decline than do measurements made near the middle of the interval. In fact, these latter measurements hardly contribute at all. A better design is to make several GFR measurements near the start and end of each observation period. I am not aware of any published results that employ this method.

Another problem, common to all clinical trials, is dealing with dropouts. Obviously they cannot be ignored, since one treatment may lead to more dropouts than another. Various techniques for dealing with dropouts have been proposed. When dropouts amount to a substantial proportion of the patients, the results of the study cannot be regarded as meaningful.

Another major problem is so-called intention-to-treat analyses. Sta-tisticians insist that the results of treatment and control groups should be analyzed separately, no matter how much overlap there is in the experi-mental variable between the two groups. Thus, for example, if a study is designed to see how blood pressure affects progression of renal disease, the actual blood pressures of the patients in the two groups are not what matters; what matters is whether a given individual has been assigned to the low–blood pressure group or the higher–blood pressure group. This means that a patient with a relatively high blood pressure who is part of the low–blood pressure group will be analyzed as if she had low blood pressure. The reason for this curious logic is that the possibility cannot be excluded that her rate of progression was slow to begin with and was scarcely influenced by the attempt to lower her blood pressure. In a secondary analysis, it can be determined in the combined patient population whether there is a relationship between blood pressure and rate of progression. But the result of this secondary analysis may be misleading: Those patients who progress the fastest, for example, may have more severe renal disease that causes higher blood pressure, rather than the blood pressure causing the progression.

Most of the published studies of progression of renal disease have been poorly controlled, often because a proper experimental design was beyond the investigators' resources. A common design, which has little to recommend it other than low cost, is a simple crossover. In this design patients are observed before and after the introduction of the experimental variable. The problem is that whatever change in progression rate (or anything else) that is observed could have taken place without the introduction of the experimental variable. Another common design is the comparison of rates of progression of two groups, one of which is treated with the experimental variable. Unless the assignment to these two groups is randomized, there may be differences between the two groups that invalidate the results. Blinding—that is, not telling the subjects which group they have been assigned to—is impossible in most diet studies but is highly desirable in drug studies. The absence of blinding leaves open the possibility that bias may affect the results.

Measuring the Quality of Life in Predialysis Patients

Recently some publications have assessed the quality of life in predialysis patients. Unfortunately, none has yet assessed the quality of life in predialysis patients on different regimens. Several publications also purport to document the "usual" biochemical abnormalities seen in predialysis patients. Again, the authors seem to forget that the results reflect the quality of care that has been provided more than the fundamental characteristics of the predialysis state.

A striking example is a series of measurements from Sweden by Stenvinkel, Heimburger, and colleagues. Their patients were assessed just before they started on dialysis, apparently never having been seen before by the investigators. At least, I hope this is the case, since the patients were clearly neglected, presumably by their physicians. Not only did they have low albumin levels, indicating malnutrition, but their bicarbonate levels were not even measured. We can assume, therefore, that acidosis (low bicarbonate level) was very common and often severe, as documented by Raymond Hakim and Michael Lazarus, who reported serum bicarbonate levels in 911 predialysis patients at Harvard. Good predialysis care can almost totally prevent low serum albumin or bicarbonate levels.

18

Dietary Treatment of the Nephrotic Syndrome

The nephrotic syndrome has been mentioned throughout the book as something that is different from kidney failure, but which often ends up causing kidney failure. Let's examine exactly what the nephrotic syndrome is and how it can be treated.

The nephrotic syndrome is defined as a very high rate of excretion of protein in the urine (greater than 3.5 g per day), a low level of albumin in the blood (less than 3.5 g per dl), and edema (swelling of soft tissues, such as the ankles, the abdomen, and around the eyes). Most patients with the nephrotic syndrome also show markedly elevated levels of cholesterol and other lipids. This condition is a form of kidney disease distinct from kidney failure. The causes are numerous, including toxic reactions to drugs, allergic reactions to bee stings, various infections, cancer, a huge list of systemic diseases, and various disorders of the heart and blood vessels. For unknown reasons, young children are often affected. Cow's milk protein intolerance is said to cause the nephrotic syndrome. It is hoped that further studies will be done on the effect on the kidney of possible allergy-inducing proteins in food. Sometimes the nephrotic syndrome disappears entirely after a few months. However, patients with the nephrotic syndrome often develop renal failure and progress to dialysis.

In the past, the low albumin concentration in the serum and the pronounced loss of protein in the urine of patients with the nephrotic syndrome led nephrologists to advise a high dietary protein intake. In the mid-1980s, however, several reports appeared documenting that dietary protein restriction not only reduced urinary loss of protein, but in some cases led to an increase in serum albumin level. As yet, no explanation for this paradoxical effect has been proposed. (Note: In these studies, most doctors used a low-protein diet instead of the supplemented very-low-protein diet that has been suggested in this book.)

Having observed serum albumin levels rise in some patients without the nephrotic syndrome when given a supplemented very-low-protein diet, my colleagues and I decided to try this regimen in patients with the nephrotic syndrome due to any cause. To our surprise we found that protein excretion decreased in all patients and serum albumin rose in most. Nevertheless, 12 of these patients who presented with glomerular filtration rates of less than 30 ml per min (about one-quarter of the normal value) eventually progressed to dialysis. The remaining 5 patients, who presented with GFRs greater than 30 ml per min, showed surprising improvement: Albumin rose to normal, cholesterol fell almost to normal, and protein excretion in the urine decreased markedly over the ensuing months. In other words, the nephrotic syndrome of these patients virtually disappeared. These changes were not the result of falling GFRs; in fact, GFRs rose in 4 of the 5 patients. Later, 4 of these 5 patients resumed a normal diet.

Subsequently, Simin Sistani and I have found that one type of nephrotic syndrome in particular benefits from this approach, a disease known as focal segmental glomerulosclerosis, which was particularly hard to treat in the past. In patients with the nephrotic syndrome, in general, the greater the amount of protein lost in the urine before starting the diet, the greater the response to diet. In fact, patients who had low amounts of protein in their urine showed no benefit from the diet, while patients with severe nephrotic syndrome usually showed a marked fall in urinary protein; only one relapsed. This finding is the opposite of conventional wisdom, which holds that patients with pronounced urinary protein are poor candidates for protein-restricted diets.

Here are some examples of people with the nephrotic syndrome who have responded to dietary treatment.

Arnold Sanderson is a retired research analyst for the Health Care Financing Administration. He was referred to Johns Hopkins one year ago with a history of hypertension for 40 years and high urinary protein for 9 years. A kidney biopsy had shown a type of glomerular disease often associated with the nephrotic syndrome called membranoproliferative glomerulonephritis. Despite a protein-restricted diet (40 g per day) and an ACE inhibitor, his serum creatinine level and the amount of protein in his urine had progressively increased. Nevertheless, he had always maintained normal levels of serum albumin and cholesterol. He had no symptoms at all, and his physical showed nothing out of order. Initially, the following results were obtained from the laboratory: serum creatinine 3.8 mg per dl, serum albumin 4.0 g per dl, GFR 26.3 ml per min, urine protein 4.8 g per day. He was placed on a very-low-protein diet supplemented by essential amino acids and has been checked every two months. Three years later, the lab data showed only moderate worsening: serum creatinine 4.7 mg per dl, serum albumin 3.8 g per dl, GFR 18.3 ml per min, urine protein 1 g per day. He remains free of symptoms. Perhaps in response to this diet, Arnold's nephrotic syndrome has stopped progressing although his kidney function has declined. His compliance with the diet has been excellent.

—Dialysis deferral: 3 years

Lavinia Leonardo is a 50-year-old resource manager for the army. She was referred to us for treatment in 1995. She had been diabetic since her second pregnancy 28 years ago. Oral antidiabetic drugs had treated the condition well until four months ago, when she needed to start on insulin injections. Ten days later she developed generalized swelling and was found to have a serum albumin level of 1.3 g per dl and urinary protein of 20 g per day. A kidney biopsy showed focal segmental glomerulosclerosis and mild diabetic glomerulosclerosis. She had been intermittently hypertensive for years and was taking an ACE inhibitor as well as other antihypertensive drugs and diuretics. She complained of fatigue, muscle cramps, swelling, and aches across the shoulders. Physical exam showed only ankle edema. Laboratory data were as follows: serum albumin 2.5 g per dl, serum cholesterol 415 mg per dl, serum creatinine 1.2 mg per dl, serum urea nitrogen 39 mg per dl*, GFR 29.8 ml per min.

Lavinia was placed on a very-low-protein diet supplemented by a double dose of essential amino acids (20 g per day). Over the next few months, her kidney disease disappeared: Her serum albumin concentration rose to normal, urine protein disappeared, and GFR rose to normal. The diet and the supplement were discontinued, and she exhibited no signs of kidney disease for the next four years.

Then, early in 2001, she developed marked protein excretion again (19 g per day) and an even more severe drop in serum albumin level (to 1.8 g per dl). Serum cholesterol rose to 340 mg per dl. Unless she consumed salt, she noted little swelling. (She was still taking diuretics plus a statin and limiting salt intake.) Resumption of the low-protein diet plus supplemental essential amino acids had little effect at first, except that serum albumin level rose slowly. By fall 2001, however, urinary protein suddenly disappeared and serum albumin level became normal. She now has no symptoms at all.

—Dialysis deferral: Permanent

Martha Blomberg is a 44-year-old office worker with the nephrotic syndrome caused by a form of glomerular disease called focal segmental glomerulosclerosis. She was first seen at Johns Hopkins in 1992. She had a very low serum albumin concentration (2.3 g per dl), pronounced urinary protein excretion (11 g per day), and high serum levels of cholesterol (340 mg per dl), LDL cholesterol (242 mg per dl), and triglycerides (294 mg per dl). These lipid abnormalities had persisted despite her taking a statin drug, pravastatin, to counteract them. Her GFR was

---

*Urea concentrations traditionally have been reported as urea nitrogen concentrations, for historical reasons; urea contains 47 percent of nitrogen by weight.

moderately reduced, 36 ml per min. When placed on a very-low-protein diet supplemented by essential amino acids, she responded slowly but profoundly: urine protein decreased over the next year to about 3 g per day, serum albumin rose to normal (3.7 g per dl), and GFR scarcely changed. By the end of 1994, the diet could be discontinued. Since then she has continued to exhibit urinary protein excretion lower than on admission (about 3 g per day), unchanging GFR, and normal serum albumin concentration. However, high blood cholesterol has continued to be a problem. During 1993 and 1994, her serum cholesterol concentration fell slowly, though not quite to normal levels, presumably as a result of the diet. But early in 1995, her liver function tests (ALT and AST) suddenly became very abnormal. Pravastatin was discontinued, and these tests returned to normal (except for a couple of unexplained lesser elevations in 1997). Serum cholesterol remained high. Tests for hepatitis were carried out and proved negative. Eventually, after much discussion and an attempt at a low-fat diet that proved ineffective, a different statin drug, atorvastatin, was started. For the first time her cholesterol levels are normal, despite continued urinary protein loss (about 1.5 g per day). We will continue to check her for liver damage from this different statin drug. Meanwhile, dialysis has been avoided, apparently permanently. Kidney function is constant after six years, and she has no symptoms on a normal diet.

—Dialysis deferral: 12 years so far

As you can see from these stories, when careful attention is paid to other health problems, a supplemented very-low-protein diet can be extremely effective in helping patients with the nephrotic syndrome avoid dialysis. Similar results were reported in preliminary form from Japan.

The means by which protein restriction improves the nephrotic syndrome are unknown. It seems curious that dietary protein restriction does not reduce protein loss in the urine in patients who lose only moderate amounts. This is the exact opposite of conventional wisdom; it is generally held that protein restriction should not be employed if there is a lot of protein in the urine.

19

Safe and Unsafe Medications for Patients with Kidney Failure

Adverse drug reactions and drug interactions are common in renal failure. Since most drugs and drug breakdown products are excreted via the kidneys, even partial loss of kidney function alters the response to a given dose. Kidney disease may change not only drug elimination, but also drug absorption and distribution throughout the body. One such effect often observed is diminished protein binding of drugs in the plasma, owing to low serum albumin level, thereby increasing the concentration of free drugs in the blood. The amount of free drug in the blood is responsible for the drug's effects. If you take a given dose of drug, the extent to which the drug gets bound to your serum albumin will have a major effect on your response: The less drug that gets bound to albumin, the greater the drug's effect on your body. Thus a lower dose of the drug may be better for you.

In other cases, a metabolic product of the administered drug is responsible for its effects. One such example is meperidine (Demerol), which is converted to normeperidine, the metabolite that combats pain; Demerol itself does not combat pain. But normeperidine can accumulate in patients with renal failure and result in seizures.

Patients with kidney failure should avoid using, if possible, two classes of drugs: nonsteroidal anti-inflammatory drugs (NSAIDs), and steroids.

Nonsteroidal Anti-inflammatory Drugs

These drugs are so called because, like adrenocortical steroids (see below), they reduce inflammation, especially in joints, but also in other tissues. NSAIDs include aspirin (also present in many over-the-counter drugs), acetaminophen (also sold as Tylenol and present in many other combination drugs), celecoxib (sold as Celebrex), ibuprofen (sold under many names, including Advil, Nuprin, and Motrin), and rofecoxib (sold as Vioxx). These are probably the most widely used drugs on the market. NSAIDs are taken for arthritic pain and for headache, among many other indications. Avoiding these pain relievers is out of the question for most people. If you do find yourself in need of a pain reliever, do not take any of these drugs for more than a few days at a time.

Long-term use of any of these drugs is likely to aggravate kidney damage and occasionally to initiate it. If you are taking any of these drugs long term, testing your urine for protein once a month or so is a good idea. If you have protein in your urine, stop the drugs and repeat the test a week or so later. If the protein is still there, tell your doctor.

Two of the most commonly used drugs, aspirin and acetaminophen, have been studied extensively to determine if they adversely affect patients with chronic kidney disease. For example, in a recent study, 918 Swedish patients with newly diagnosed kidney failure and 980 control subjects were asked about their prior consumption of these drugs. The people with kidney disease reported taking both drugs two and a half times more frequently than the controls, suggesting that these drugs may have aggravated kidney disease. Some people (in both groups) reported a lifetime consumption that totaled more than 50 pounds, which sounds unbelievable but is not really extraordinary; taking a few pills every day for several decades adds up. However, the study's authors could not find hard evidence that the drugs had *caused* kidney disease.

It is interesting to note, however, that there was no association between kidney disease and the use of other analgesics, such as propoxyphene (Darvon), nonsteroidal drugs other than aspirin (such as naproxyn, sold as Aleve, among other brands), codeine, or pyrazolones (generally not available in the United States). The implication is that these other drugs are safer for pain in people with kidney disease, but this inference must be considered preliminary.

The newer so-called Cox-2 inhibitors, Celebrex and Vioxx, may or may not be preferable. Although they have been widely advertised as less likely to cause gastric irritation, this claim is questionable. Whether these drugs have any adverse effect on the progression of renal failure has not yet been established, but since they do not cause acute kidney damage, or at least not often, they may be relatively safe. They do, however, raise blood pressure a little and may increase the likelihood of heart disease slightly (especially Vioxx) when taken long term. It is not advisable to take these drugs chronically either.

A possible alternative for treatment of arthritic or rheumatic pain in patients with chronic kidney disease is salicyl salicylate, sold as Disalcid. This drug may not activate the pathways that lead to kidney damage; however, my experience with this drug is quite limited.

Steroids

The term "steroids" is used loosely for a large group of drugs that act like the hormones that affect carbohydrate metabolism. They are known as stress hormones, because their production by the adrenal cortex increases in response to stress. The term "steroids" is actually a misnomer, because a number of other substances in the body have similar chemical structure and also can be called steroids, such as vitamin D. The many drugs on the market referred to loosely as "steroids" differ in absorbability, speed of action, potency, and relative strength. These drugs are most often taken as anti-inflammatory agents. In fact, a Nobel Prize was awarded for this discovery in the treatment of arthritis. They are also used to suppress allergic symptoms. All these drugs have a number of side effects, especially in large doses. Some of the drugs in this category are: cortisol, cortisone, dexamethasone, hydrocortisone, prednisolone, prednisone, triamicinolone, and many others. These are chemical names; there are innumerable trade names.

High doses of steroids are used therapeutically in certain renal diseases, with some success but also with moderately severe side effects. In some patients with renal failure, the oral administration or injection of steroids can accelerate disease progression and should be avoided. Also, it is important to note that steroids increase protein turnover and blunt the mechanisms that permit the body to conserve protein in response to a low-protein diet; thus patients who chronically take steroids should not consume low-protein diets. "Topical" steroids—steroid-containing creams, ointments, eyedrops, and nasal sprays—are not harmful to the kidneys unless used in very large amounts or for prolonged periods.

Because of the likelihood that over-the-counter medicines might react with prescription medications, always consult your pharmacist or your doctor to get advice on what might be best for you to take.

20

Transplantation as an Alternative to Dialysis

The first kidney transplant was performed in 1954, at Peter Bent Brigham Hospital in Boston by Dr. Joseph E. Murray, from one identical twin to another. In 1990 Dr. Murray shared the Nobel Prize with another transplant pioneer, Dr. E. Donnall Thomas, who was the first to perform a successful transplant of bone marrow. In the decades since these first transplants, we've learned much about how to prevent rejection of transplanted organs, and kidney transplantation has become a good alternative to dialysis.

If you have progressed to end-stage renal disease (ESRD), a kidney transplant may be the preferred treatment for you. Transplantation has even been recommended to infants, elderly patients, diabetic patients, and those with other significant health problems who would not have been candidates in the past. A kidney transplant offers improved quality of life over both kinds of dialysis. Patients who do well after transplantation generally report improvement in vitality and freedom to return to the style of life that they experienced before their progression to ESRD.

A successful transplant takes a coordinated effort of a whole health-care team, including your nephrologist, transplant surgeon, transplant coordinator, pharmacist, dietitian, and social worker. But you and your family are the most important members of your healthcare team. By learning about your treatment, you can work with your healthcare team to give yourself the best possible results, and you can lead a full, active life.

What a Kidney Transplant Involves

Kidney transplantation involves placing a healthy kidney from another person into your body. This one kidney takes over the work of your two failed kidneys. Before transplantation can be considered, your physicians need to determine if you are healthy enough to undergo the surgery. Cancer or other significant diseases might make transplantation unlikely to succeed. During the transplant, the surgeon places the new kidney inside your lower abdomen and connects the artery and vein of the new kidney to your artery and vein. Your blood flows through the new kidney, which makes urine and regulates your bodily content of many substances, just as your own kidneys did when they were healthy. Often the new kidney will start making urine as soon as blood starts flowing through it, but sometimes as long as a few days may pass before it starts working. Unless they are causing infection or high blood pressure, your own kidneys are left in place. Most people remain in the hospital just a few days after a kidney transplant.

Your body's immune system is designed to keep you healthy by sensing foreign invaders and rejecting them. After your surgery, your immune system will sense that your new kidney is foreign. To keep your body from rejecting it, you'll have to take drugs that turn off or suppress your immune response. These drugs have a large list of unfortunate side effects, including a slight risk of developing cancer. Even if you do everything you're supposed to do, your body still may reject the new kidney and you may need to go back on dialysis. That said, odds are good for transplants. The one-year survival of transplanted kidneys has improved dramatically: It is now greater than 90 percent, mainly because of better drugs used to suppress rejection. Patient deaths in the first year after transplantation are uncommon and are due to the usual causes seen in people without kidney transplants. However, the longer you wait on dialysis for a transplant, the greater the chance of the transplant failing.

Undergoing a transplant without first having been in dialysis is uncommon, for several reasons:

1. There is the is the possibility that waiting too long may impair the health of the recipient to the point that the risk of complications increases.

2. Transplantation entails the use of immunosuppressive drugs, which have a very small but distinct risk of causing malignancy (particularly lymphomas).

3. The establishment of a satisfactory vascular or peritoneal access for the dialysis procedure makes starting dialysis easier.

None of these reasons, however, is compelling. They must be weighed against the risk of dialysis itself (which entails a greater than 20 percent annual mortality), as well as the possibility that once a patient is started on dialysis, the search for a donor loses some of its urgency.

Medicare pays most of the costs of transplantation (to both recipient and donor). Medicare recoups the initially higher costs of transplantation within three years, because of the high cost of dialysis.

Sources of Donor Kidneys

Most transplanted kidneys come from people who have died, but there are not enough of these potential donors to meet the needs. A growing number of transplanted kidneys now come from living family members or friends. Most people can donate a kidney with little risk.

The advantages of a living donor are:

- The waiting period is eliminated.

- Kidneys from family members are more likely to be good matches.

- Kidneys from living donors don't need to be transported from one site to another.

- Living donation helps people on the waiting list for cadaveric kidneys by shortening the list.

Before donating a kidney, the donor needs thorough medical evaluation and must be evaluated to see if he or she is a good match. Suitability formerly depended on blood type (A, B, AB, or O) and other genetic markers called HLA factors. A higher number of matching factors seemed to increase the chances that the kidney would last for a long time.

Gradually these limitations have been circumvented, and now almost anyone can give a kidney to anyone else. Nevertheless, the prospective donor's blood is mixed with the patient's blood to see if a reaction occurs, which could be caused by antibodies.

The donor and the recipient are operated on at the same time, usually in side-by-side rooms. Most living donor surgery is now done through a small incision penetrated by an instrument called a laporoscope, through which the surgeon can see the donor's kidney and its blood vessels; the kidney is removed through a small incision. This means that postoperative incisional pain, which was formerly a prolonged complaint in many donors, is now almost nonexistent. A donor's average hospitalization is only 66 hours, and the risk of overall mortality is about 0.03 percent. Originally, doctors anticipated a long-term decline in the function of the remaining kidney, but there is no compelling evidence of that occurring. In fact, for unknown reasons, donation may improve the donor's quality of life and even life expectancy. Health insurance remains available for kidney donors. Age is no contraindication for kidney donation: Healthy grandparents are an excellent source for young patients. Children and mentally incompetent persons can also be donors, in theory, although this is widely felt to be unacceptable, because of the impossibility of informed consent. Financial rewards for giving a kidney have generally been disparaged in the United States, though there are dissenting voices.

In 2000 Michael M. Abecassis, speaking for a steering committee chosen from national organizations, issued a consensus statement concerning live organ donors: "The person who gives consent to be a live organ donor should be competent, willing to donate, free from coercion, medically and psychosocially suitable, fully informed of the risks and benefits as a donor, and fully informed of the risks, benefits and alternative treatment available to the recipient. The benefits to both donor and recipient must outweigh the risks associated with the donation and transplantation of the living donor organ."

The trouble with this statement is that it overlooks the possibility of "nondirected" kidney donation, that is, giving a kidney without knowing who the recipient may be. In a recent survey, a surprising fraction of the U.S. population expressed willingness to give a kidney without payment to someone they didn't know. Of course, many of these individuals might change their minds when faced with the reality. The detailed finances of this process remain to be worked out; clearly the donors should not incur significant expenses, but equally clearly, they should not receive a monetary reward for giving up a part of their anatomy.

For physicians, the main problem with this process is that it violates one of the precepts of the Hippocratic Oath, namely, first and foremost to do no harm. When a nondirected kidney is removed, the donor incurs a small but real risk, for which the only corresponding benefit is the pleasure of altruism. This makes most surgeons uncomfortable, and they suspect that the donor is emotionally unstable. Most transplant surgeons prefer that the donor should be emotionally close to the recipient.

Paying for a kidney (as has been done in recent years in several third-world countries) can lead to adverse consequences. In Iran, a questionnaire was recently sent to 100 kidney donors. Ninety percent did not know the recipients. Money was the principal motivation for donation in 97 percent of them. Yet three-quarters concluded that kidney sale should be banned. Half of them stated that they "hated" the recipients, and 82 percent were dissatisfied with their own behavior.

By contrast, donating a kidney, without payment, to a known recipient (friend or relative) has a strongly positive psychological impact. Unfortunately, many U.S. transplant centers do not actively encourage donations from spouses or friends, and a majority would not consider an altruistic stranger. Perhaps these attitudes will change.

21

When to Opt
for Dialysis

Despite all the work that you may have done in following the advice and treatment plans given in this book, and working with dietitians and your doctors, you may find that one day you do need dialysis. When kidney function gets very low, dialysis is necessary to replace the work of healthy kidneys and to remove waste products from the blood and body fluids. The two types of dialysis, hemodialysis and peritoneal dialysis, are very different.

Hemodialysis

During hemodialysis treatment, your blood travels through tubes into a dialyzer, which filters out wastes and extra water. Then the cleaned blood flows through another set of tubes back into your body. The dialyzer is connected to a machine that monitors blood flow and removes wastes from the blood. Patients usually need hemodialysis three times a week, with each treatment lasting from three to five or more hours. During treatment you can read, write, sleep, or watch TV. Several months before your first treatment, an access to your bloodstream must be created in the wrist. You may need to stay overnight in the hospital, but many patients have this procedure done on an outpatient basis. This access provides an efficient way for the blood to be carried from your body to the dialysis machine and back without causing discomfort. The two main types of access are a fistula, in which an artery is connected directly to a vein, and a graft, which connects an artery to a vein with a synthetic tube. When you go in for your regular dialysis, you're given a local anesthetic and then your blood is drawn out with a needle from that access point.

Problems with these forms of access are the most common reason for hospitalization among people on hemodialysis. They include infection, blockage by clots, and poor blood flow. You may need to undergo repeated surgeries in order to get a properly functioning access. Other problems can be caused by rapid changes during dialysis in your body's water and chemical balance. Muscle cramps and sudden drop in blood pressure, which can make you weak, dizzy, or nauseated, are common.

Peritoneal Dialysis

Peritoneal dialysis uses the lining of your abdominal organs to filter your blood. This lining, called the peritoneal membrane, acts like an artificial kidney. A dialysis solution of minerals and sugar (dextrose) travels through a soft tube into your abdomen. The dextrose draws wastes, chemicals, and extra water from the tiny blood vessels in your peritoneal membrane through the membrane and into the dialysis solution. After several hours, the used solution is drained from your abdomen through the tube, taking the wastes from your blood with it. Then your abdomen is filled with a fresh dialysis solution, and the cycle is repeated.

Before your first treatment, a surgeon places a small soft tube called a catheter into your abdomen. The catheter tends to work better if there is adequate time (usually from 10 to 20 days) for the insertion site to heal. This catheter stays there permanently.

There are three varieties of peritoneal dialysis: continuous ambulatory peritoneal dialysis, continuous cycler-assisted peritoneal dialysis (which requires a machine), and a combination of the two. Patients usually can perform peritoneal dialysis at home without assistance.

The most common problem with peritoneal dialysis is peritonitis, a serious abdominal infection. This infection can occur if the opening where the catheter enters your body becomes infected or if contamination occurs as the catheter is connected and disconnected. The treatment is antibiotics.

When Should You Start Dialysis?

In my opinion, many people are started on dialysis too early in their kidney failure. Dialysis should be avoided as long as possible. In recent years, doctors have begun starting patients on dialysis earlier and earlier, in the hope of thereby reducing some of the complications of dialysis. Because it has been demonstrated repeatedly that late referral by a primary care doctor to a nephrologist increases the subsequent morbidity and mortality of patients, some doctors have inferred that patients who see a nephrologist earlier and go on dialysis sooner will fare better.

Not so. The issue has been obscured by the fact that late referral to a nephrologist often means urgent initiation of dialysis, which is well known to increase death rates. In fact, when patients who are already under a nephrologist's care are started on dialysis late (that is, with relatively advanced kidney failure) are compared with those started earlier (that is, with relatively mild kidney failure), no difference in mortality has been demonstrated.

Predialysis care is considerably safer than dialysis. Furthermore, patients approaching dialysis who have not been told about the dietary treatment plan (as outlined in this book) should be told that this option can safely defer dialysis for an average of a year. Failure to inform patients of this alternative treatment is indefensible.

It is often assumed that dialysis makes people feel better. But this is not always the case. Birgitta Klang and Naomi Clyne in Stockholm measured perceived well-being and functional capacity in 28 patients before and after starting dialysis. They found that, after starting dialysis, fatigue, lack of energy, and functional disability in work increased.

It is also widely assumed that dialysis improves objective measures of kidney disease. These measures can be summarized by the scoring method given in Chapter 5. Obviously when a person whose score is very low is placed on dialysis, he or she is going to achieve a higher score, because the patient is no longer being neglected. Attributing this improvement to dialysis is unjustified. When a person whose score is already very high is placed on dialysis, his or her score cannot improve. This dilemma is hard to resolve. There is no easy way to find out just what starting dialysis does to objective measures of kidney disease.

In my opinion, dialysis should never be undertaken unless the symptoms are sufficiently severe that they will be improved by dialysis. As noted in other chapters, severe fatigue, muscle cramps, and shortness of breath may occur as kidney failure reaches the end stage. Another complication of severe kidney failure that may precipitate dialysis is inflammation of the covering of the heart, the pericardium. This causes severe chest pain and also may aggravate heart failure, and can be treated only by dialysis. As you approach the end stage, you will need to be closely monitored with respect to these symptoms. Obviously this will require you to see your doctor every week or so, but predialysis care is considerably safer than dialysis.

Establishing any benefit to starting dialysis earlier will require a randomized study. It also will require that predialysis mortality be at least comparable to dialysis mortality, which seems highly unlikely.

One of the most consistent advocates of early dialysis published a study comparing mortality on dialysis in two groups of patients: those started at a serum creatinine concentration of less than 10 mg per dl versus those started at a serum creatinine concentration of greater than 10. No difference in mortality during the ensuing 60 months was seen. Perhaps the most striking feature of this study is that the two survival curves are just as close in the first year as they are thereafter. In other words, patients starting dialysis at a serum creatinine level under 10 mg per dl began to die within the first few months. Since this was not a randomized comparison, it fails to validate early or late dialysis.

What is certain is that the mortality of dialysis is many times greater than the mortality of predialysis care. Three studies have now been reported in which the mortality of predialysis care is documented; all three report a predialysis mortality of close to 2.5 percent per year. These studies cannot be definitive, since predialysis mortality obviously will increase as renal failure progresses, especially if dialysis is deferred too long. If dialysis is deferred indefinitely, mortality of predialysis is obviously 100 percent. National statistics give the mortality of people on dialysis as approximately 23 percent per year.

One of the most remarkable policies recently recommended by some nephrologists is to start dialysis if a patient's protein intake falls. It has been known for decades that people with kidney failure tend to shun meat and other high-protein foods as their renal insufficiency progresses, though the explanation of this long-standing observation is not known. It is also well known that protein deficiency, manifested by low serum albumin concentration, is a bad prognostic sign for people starting dialysis; it predicts shorter survival. These nephrologists have put these two observations together and inferred that anyone whose renal failure is so bad that they shun meat must be in danger of developing protein deficiency and should therefore be started on dialysis forthwith.

The problem here is that the nephrologists are overlooking other highly relevant observations. Most important, it has been well established that the only way to prevent low serum albumin concentration in patients approaching ESRD is to restrict dietary protein severely and to add a supplement of essential amino acids (or their keto-analogues), as I have emphasized repeatedly in this book. The progressively falling intake of meat by patients approaching the end stage is accompanied by progressive loss of appetite and falling caloric intake. The fall in serum albumin concentration is attributable in part to low caloric intake and in part to inflammatory processes of unknown origin. Whatever these inflammatory processes may be, they seem to be prevented by a supplemented very-low-protein diet.

Dr. William E. Mitch, a well-known nephrologist, has put it well: "Evidence that dietary protein spontaneously decreases in progressively uremic patients should not be construed as an argument against the use of dietary therapy. Rather, it is a persuasive argument to restrict dietary protein in order to minimize [chronic renal failure] complications while preserving nutritional status. In patients with uremia or progression despite other measures, dietary therapy should be started along with monitoring for dietary compliance and nutritional adequacy."

The tacit assumption that an increase in protein intake will improve protein nutrition has never been confirmed experimentally, even though this experiment could be easily performed. A more probable result of higher meat intake is further loss of appetite, perhaps with nausea and vomiting, and a further decrease in caloric intake, thus aggravating malnutrition and reducing serum albumin concentration even further.

Placing a patient on dialysis because he or she spontaneously consumes a relatively small amount of protein is utter folly. The "wisdom of the body" in this instance is greater than the wisdom of the physician. How this cockeyed theory could have been incorporated into the official guidelines for managing renal failure, promulgated by the National Kidney Foundation, is an interesting question. The chairman of this committee was J. D. Kopple, who also is a coauthor of a 1999 editorial "Should Protein Intake Be Restricted in Pre-Dialysis Patients?" that concludes "with rare exceptions, patients with CRF [chronic renal failure] should receive a trial of a protein-restricted diet before being started on dialysis." It is difficult to understand how Dr. Kopple could reconcile these two divergent views.

Physicians like me who work with predialysis patients and try to defer or avoid dialysis are vulnerable to being accused of waiting too long before starting dialysis and thus putting our patients in jeopardy in some ill-defined way. In order to escape this charge, I have been obliged to adopt the following policy: I have made *none* of the decisions to initiate dialysis (or transplantation) in my current series of patients; the patient's chosen dialysis (or transplant) physician made all these decisions.

Sometimes these decisions are made by one of the local teams here at Johns Hopkins, in which case their decisions are usually soundly based. But when the decision is made elsewhere, the patient sometimes encounters difficult and prolonged arguments. A major difficulty for predialysis patients may be persuading nephrologists to defer dialysis until symptoms clearly indicate it. On the other hand, a few of my patients have become so convinced of the value of dietary therapy or so much in denial that they defer dialysis too long and develop complications.

Remember, it's your body and your choice. You can solicit opinions from your healthcare team, but it's your body and you know best how it's doing. There is an inherent conflict between wanting to cooperate with and trust the physician who will be in charge of your future care and wanting to avoid unnecessary risk. Every patient approaching end-stage kidney disease faces this challenge.

The Withholding and Withdrawal of Dialysis

Two other topics need to be addressed, unpleasant though they are: withholding of dialysis and withdrawal from dialysis. Either is fatal within a few weeks.

Withholding dialysis obviously comes up for discussion only when the burdens of dialysis treatment are expected to exceed its benefits. It is not hard to imagine circumstances under which this could be true. Dementia, multisystem disease including cancer, and extreme old age come to mind. In the early days of chronic dialysis, people over a certain age were automatically refused government-subsidized dialysis in Great Britain and other countries, and this issue keeps coming up. For a time people with diabetes were turned down. Present practice in the United States is to accept just about anybody. Clearly some of the people being placed on dialysis cannot be expected to receive much benefit from it.

Withdrawal from dialysis, which is an even thornier issue, is very common. As noted earlier, the official U.S. government report for 1999 on dialysis nationwide states that "1 in 5 patients withdraws from dialysis before death." Many other publications confirm this. Sometimes the reasons are understandable, but sometimes people just want to quit. The appropriate response for the physician is not always obvious. In general, first the patient's mental competence is assessed. Then the patient's "surrogate," meaning a next of kin or someone else designated as a decision maker for the patient, is consulted. The surrogate may (and often does) disagree with the patient's decision. The courts may get involved. If dialysis continues, and at some later date the patient expresses gratitude, everyone agrees that continuance was the right decision. But this may not occur.

If you do have to go on dialysis, you may want to read *Kidney Failure: The Facts*, by Dr. Stewart Cameron, a distinguished British nephrologist, published by Oxford University Press in 1996. Although it is out of print, you may be able to get it through your library. It is far and away the best book for patients on this topic.

The question of when to start dialysis and whether to try to postpone it by dietary treatment will never be settled until someone completes a study in which patients are assigned by chance to start dialysis early or to try to defer it by dietary therapy. Such a study has begun in Italy, comparing the survival on dialysis of two groups of elderly patients with end-stage kidney disease: One group was started on dialysis late (average creatinine clearance only 3.9 ml per min, considerably lower than the average creatinine clearance at the start of dialysis in the United States), after an average of 14 months on a supplemented very-low-protein diet; the other group was started directly on dialysis (average creatinine clearance 6.7 ml per min). So far, in the first group, 60 percent were still alive after 4.6 years of dialysis; in the second group, all had died by that time. This finding seems to suggest that predialysis treatment with a low-protein diet improves long-term survival.

A second trial has been started in Italy by the same group, in which older patients who meet the accepted U.S. criteria for starting dialysis are assigned by chance either to start dialysis (at one of several centers) or to undertake a very-low-protein diet supplemented by a mixture of ketoacids and amino acids. The latter group is then followed until dialysis becomes necessary, and the long-term outcome of the two groups is compared.

An immediate problem for the doctors planning this trial is: What are the criteria that make dialysis necessary in those on diet therapy?

I have examined the criteria proposed by these researchers. Clearly they are very sensitive to any possible criticism that they may be withholding dialysis in patients on dietary therapy.

A simple and generally useful criterion for starting dialysis is the presence of symptoms that can be expected to improve on dialysis. This criterion would exclude high blood potassium (which can always be treated; see Chapter 12) and almost every instance of hypertension (almost always, a combination of drugs will lower blood pressure into the desired range; see Chapter 9). Others have included "intractable" acidosis; this simply means that the patient has not consumed enough alkali (see Chapter 10). (Sodium retention secondary to alkali administration can always be treated by diuretics.)

22

Patients Who Have Avoided Dialysis

Here are stories of some patients who came to see me or contacted me regarding their kidney failure. I have recommended dietary treatment to all of them who were symptomatic and offered others the opportunity to start dietary treatment as well, after explaining that there was no evidence that it helped in the presymptomatic stage. (A few wanted to try it anyway.) As you will see by reading in particular the story of Leigh Dell, all of this can be done by telephone and does not require people to come to Johns Hopkins. About 5 percent of patients referred to me have declined to try a very-low-protein diet.

I hope these stories will inspire you to consider the recommendations set forth in this book to improve your treatment and your health.

Patients with Diabetes

Marshall Wynngarden, a 34-year-old physician, came to Johns Hopkins in 1986, with a history of insulin-dependent diabetes since age 9 and renal failure since 1983. He was complaining of fatigue, arthritic pains, sexual dysfunction, and muscle cramps. Despite an ACE inhibitor and moderate protein restriction, his kidney function declined. In 1988 he was started on a very-low-protein diet, supplemented by amino acids alternating with ketoacids. Symptoms improved, but he continued to have difficulty with control of his diabetes. Kidney function continued to decline slowly, and he finally decided to start dialysis in 1992, after four years.

—Dialysis deferral: 4 years

See also Larry Phee (p.133) and Eve Magee (p.132)

Patients with Kidney Disease Secondary to Obstructed Outflow of Urine (Interstitial Nephritis)

Ernie Ball is a computer systems analyst. When he was 38, he visited his doctor because he had pain in his flanks. A urine test showed protein plus red cells, and his doctor told him that he had a urinary tract infection and urethral stricture. Leg swelling appeared soon thereafter. He had taken analgesics (aspirin or Anacin plus Dristan) daily for years because of headaches. By age 40, he had high blood pressure and signs of moderately severe kidney failure. At age 56, by which time his serum creatinine concentration was 6.4 mg per dl, indicating severe kidney failure, he started a supplemented very-low-protein diet. He succeeded in deferring dialysis for four more years by means of a very-low-protein, low-salt diet plus either amino acids or ketoacids, antihypertensive drugs, diuretics, calcium, zinc, iron, vitamins, and sodium polystyrene sulfonate.

—Dialysis deferral: 4 years

Jason Bardereck, a 41-year-old production manager, had been diagnosed with a kidney disease called IgA nephropathy four years previously, after protein was noted in his urine on a routine checkup. Since two years ago, serum creatinine had been elevated (1.7 mg/dl rising to 3.5 mg/dl) and he had hypertension, treated with various drugs, most recently the combination of pindolol (a beta sympathetic blocker), amlodopine (a calcium channel blocker), and furosemide (a diuretic). A month ago he quit smoking, and for one month he has been taking fish oil. He had had virtually no symptoms until a few days before entry, when he first noted muscle cramps at night and ankle swelling.

Physical exam showed blood pressure 150/88, heart rate 56/min, and ankle edema.

Pindolol and amlodopine were discontinued and he was started on a combination of lisinopril (an ACE inhibitor) and hydrochlorothiazide (a diuretic).

Blood pressure remained high despite diuresis, so minoxidil (a vasodilator), metolazone (a diuretic), and atenolol (a beta blocker) were substituted. Blood pressure finally came under control.

GFR, initially measured at about 30 ml/min, gradually decreased to 14 ml/min as serum creatinine rose to 5.5 mg/dl, but both GFR and serum creatinine have scarcely changed in the past year since adding ketoconazole, 200 mg/day. He has no symptoms and continues to work full time.

—Dialysis deferral: 5 years so far

Another example of avoidance of dialysis for several years with the aid of a supplemented very-low-protein diet is Mory East, a 32-year-old physician. At age 10, he developed recurrent fevers and was found to have defects in the ureters, which drain urine from each kidney into the bladder. These defects limited the outflow of urine from his kidneys and led to frequent urinary tract infections. He was operated on at that time, and the ureters were reimplanted into the bladder. Afterward he did better but had continuing protein in his urine, showing that his kidneys had been damaged. Two years ago X rays of the kidneys, after dye injection, showed that the drainage systems on both sides were dilated by the back pressure from the bladder. His kidney function had fallen to about half of normal. As his function continued to deteriorate, further surgery was performed on both sides to improve outflow. By this time he noted some fatigue but had no other symptoms. Physical exam was negative except for mild hypertension. His first glomerular filtration rate (GFR) at Johns Hopkins was 24.3 ml per min, or about one-quarter of normal. He had moderate acidosis (CO_2 18 mM) and high serum potassium (6.3 mEq per liter). Serum creatinine was 3.0 mg per dl, serum urea nitrogen 36 mg per dl, and urine protein 1.1 g per day. For about one year, he was followed with periodic GFR tests, while receiving a low-protein diet (0.6 g per kg per day), sodium bicarbonate, an ACE inhibitor, and a beta-blocker. An alpha-blocker was substituted for the ACE inhibitor because his blood pressure was not well controlled. Sodium polystyrene sulfonate was added intermittently to lower his serum potassium level. Because some progressive loss of kidney function was detected, in January 1989 he was started on a very-low-protein diet (0.3 g per kg per day) supplemented (initially) by essential amino acids. For the next four years he followed the same diet and took alternately essential amino acids or ketoacids (mostly the latter). His GFR declined very slowly during this period, finally reaching 5.84 ml per minute at the end of 1993, with his serum creatinine rising to 13.4 mg per dl. Nevertheless, his serum urea nitrogen was only 39 mg per dl, reflecting his excellent compliance with the diet (which reduces urea formation). Serum albumin concentration remained normal (greater than 4 g per dl). During this four-year period he and his wife felt sufficiently optimistic to adopt a baby boy. He finally went on dialysis at the start of 1994, by which time he was complaining of intermittent nausea, occasional vomiting, itching, forgetfulness (but no drowsiness, confusion, or lethargy), and mild shortness of breath on exertion. Thus he probably deferred dialysis for about four years.

—Dialysis deferral: 4 years

Harry Eichhorn, a 78-year-old retired army general, was referred to me eight years ago. He had had high blood pressure since age 40,which may have been a contributor to his kidney failure. Another possible cause of his kidney failure was Motrin, one of many analgesics that can damage the kidneys when taken for prolonged periods. He took Motrin daily from 1976 to 1984 for arthritis. Protein was detected in his urine in 1985, and red cells in 1986. He was taking drugs for hypertension, a drug for high serum cholesterol, and diuretics. The only symptom he would admit to was mild fatigue. His course was complicated by the development of a form of malignancy of the bone marrow (a mono- clonal gammopathy), for which he received a number of short courses of treatment with high doses of steroids, and also by the development of prostate cancer, successfully treated by surgery. He has some diffi- culty in following a low-protein diet, but at least avoids high-protein foods, and takes essential amino acids. He switched from Motrin to Disalcid. Kidney function continued to decline at about 3 ml per minute per year. Nevertheless, he still plays 18 holes of golf without a cart. His last measurement of kidney function (on June 17, 2002) came back as 8.7 ml per minute, or less than 10 percent of normal. Fatigue got worse and he finally started dialysis in September 2002.

—Dialysis deferral: 7 years

Patients with Kidney Failure Caused by Drug Abuse

Leigh Dell, age 73, has never been to Johns Hopkins, because he lives too far away. He has had protein in his urine for many years (perhaps as a result of taking Advil over a period of years following a leg fracture). He learned in August 1999 that his serum creatinine level was elevated (to 2.9 mg per dl) and his serum urea nitrogen level was 58 mg per dl (normal is less than 25 mg per dl). His wife, after some reading, decided to start a low-protein diet and tried to assemble an essential amino acid mixture from individual amino acids sold at the health food store. A renal dietitian they saw told him to discard the amino acids and to eat 60 g per day of protein. His serum creatinine increased to 4.1 mg per dl. His wife located a complete mixture of essential amino acids (Nutramine) and also put him on a 23 g protein diet. His energy increased markedly, and he managed to lose weight. They found a nephrologist, who advised against the program they were following and recommended that he instead take 70 g of dietary protein per day. The nephrologist also said that Leigh should get ready for dialysis. However, the couple persisted with dietary treatment.

By October 29, 2002, Leigh's serum creatinine level was back down to 3.5 mg per dl and his serum urea nitrogen level was 32 mg per dl. Serum albumin level is normal (3.9 g per dl). His nephrologist now tells him that it may be possible that he will never need dialysis. Leigh is currently consuming between 40 and 50 g of protein per day and taking 10.5 g of amino acids per day. He has no symptoms, and plays tennis, gardens, and goes to the gym.

—Dialysis deferral: 5 years so far

Tim Ahlstrom first came to Johns Hopkins in March 1989, at age 50, with the following history. Protein had been noted in his urine during a routine exam 25 years earlier. Four years earlier he had developed heart failure, fever, anemia, and a moderate degree of kidney failure, all of which remained unexplained and receded, except for the kidney failure, which persisted. He was placed on a diet mildly restricted in protein and given drugs to control high blood pressure. He gained 30 to 40 pounds in the next two years, but then decided to do something about his health. He quit his three-pack-a-day smoking habit and, six months before coming to Johns Hopkins, quit alcohol too. He managed to lose 45 pounds. The recurrent headaches for which he had been taking at least 4 aspirin tablets daily for 30 years receded. He started a regular exercise program. At about this time he saw a kidney specialist, who told him that he should start thinking about dialysis and/or transplantation and that there was nothing he could do to prevent end-stage kidney failure, probably by summer 1989. Tim did some reading in the medical library and made an appointment at Johns Hopkins.

On arrival here his blood pressure was alarmingly high (215/100), kidney function was 15 percent of normal, and blood chemical values were moderately abnormal. The dietitian instructed him on a very-low-protein diet (0.3 g per kg, or 33 g per day), to be supplemented with essential amino acids and later alternately with ketoacids. His blood pressure eventually came down to normal and, after a year, his kidney function actually improved. At about this time he decided to write a book about his experiences with kidney disease, which was published in 1991 *(The Kidney Patient's Book)*. This remarkable book tells how Tim learned of the alternatives available to patients with kidney failure, what the outcomes of dialysis and transplantation are for patients at differing ages, and how to follow a low-protein diet. He published this book himself and, with the aid of his daughter Susan, kept spreading the word, despite having reached the end stage and starting dialysis in April 1992.

Tim died a few years later. He had made contact with virtually every prominent nephrologist in the field and with every governmental and nongovernmental agency involved in kidney disease, and had attended and presented papers in the United States and abroad on nutrition and kidney disease. Tim was a prime example of a patient taking charge of his own illness. I urge you to read his book. In the words of Dr. Arnold S. Relman, former editor of the *New England Journal of Medicine*, it is "an interesting and understandable discussion for kidney patients that does not compromise medical accuracy or objectivity."

—Dialysis deferral: 3 years

Patients with Polycystic Kidney Disease

Doris Balboni, a 67-year-old retired nurse with polycystic kidney disease, was found to have severe renal failure, with a glomerular filtration rate of 10.2 ml per minute and a serum creatinine concentration of 4.2 mg per dl. She was placed on a very-low-protein diet supplemented alternately by an essential amino acid mixture and by a ketoacid/amino acid mixture, both devoid of tryptophan. (Tryptophan was omitted because the Food and Drug Administration had decreed that it could not be used as a dietary supplement until the cause of a severe form of muscle disease, related to one particular commercial source of tryptophan, was clarified.) Serum tryptophan concentration fell, reaching a low of 4.16 uM (normal is 34 to 66 uM—this may be the lowest ever recorded). Serum transferrin concentration and albumin concentration also fell progressively, becoming distinctly subnormal by six months. At this point Doris was clearly suffering from clinical protein deficiency caused by lack of tryptophan. She was complaining of fatigue and loss of appetite (but not clearly more so than before). There was no increase in body weight, but ankle swelling appeared (which could also have been caused by her starting nifedipine, see page 105). After six months, tryptophan capsules (200 or 400 mg per day) were started with no other changes in her regimen. Before this was done, and again two months later, she underwent detailed neuropsychological testing. Serum transferrin concentration rose promptly, and later serum albumin concentration also rose to normal. Serum tryptophan scarcely changed until four months had passed, at which point it rose rapidly into the normal range. There was no change in neuropsychological tests with tryptophan repletion (despite the fact that tryptophan deficiency has been said to cause brain dysfunction). Doris managed to postpone dialysis for another year while on the same regimen, thus deferring dialysis for a total of 20 months. Clearly progression of her renal failure was very slow.

—Dialysis deferral: 2 years

Ella Johnson, a 49-year-old school teacher, came to Johns Hopkins in 1994. Polycystic kidney disease had been diagnosed from an abdominal scan four years earlier, although it was not seen in an X ray of the kidneys at age 22. The X ray was performed because she had recurrent urinary tract infections ever since age 18 and had required urethral dilatations. High blood pressure had been present for nine years and had been treated with a variety of drugs, including an ACE inhibitor. She had no symptoms of kidney failure. Her mother had had polycystic kidney disease too and had been a patient here. Ella had two healthy children. Physical exam was normal except that the left kidney could be felt easily and was therefore considerably enlarged.

At her request, despite the absence of symptoms, she was placed on a very-low-protein diet supplemented by essential amino acids. She also started fish oil and gets regular exercise. She does not smoke. During nine years of follow-up, she has progressed very slowly (1.8 ml per minute per year). At this rate she will be well into her 70s before she needs dialysis or transplantation.

—Dialysis deferral: 10 years

Patients with Hypertensive Kidney Disease

Chester Land, a black retired postal supervisor, was referred at age 61 with a 20-year history of hypertension. By age 59 his serum creatinine level was elevated, though he had no symptoms of kidney disease. Physical exam showed only hypertension, but kidney function was severely reduced. He was prescribed a very-low-protein diet supplemented by essential amino acids or ketoacids (in addition to his antihypertensive drugs and diuretics). A few years later a routine lab report raised the spectre of severe intestinal bleeding, until the lab error was discovered. At age 66 a blood test for prostate cancer was reported as abnormal and confirmed by prostate biopsy. He underwent a course of radiotherapy. During eight years of dietary treatment, kidney function did not worsen; nevertheless, he eventually started dialysis. Despite some complications, he is still doing fairly well, having received a transplant. In retrospect, dietary treatment probably deferred dialysis for about four years.

—Dialysis deferral: 4 years

A striking example is Lynne Bright, a 39-year-old secretary at a clinical laboratory in Indiana, who came to Johns Hopkins in February 2000. Two years earlier she had learned that she had kidney failure, when a routine exam revealed an elevated serum creatinine. At that time she had already had high blood pressure for about a year. Urine protein was also abnormal (3 g per day) but serum albumin concentration was normal. She had felt tired for about seven months, but denied loss of appetite, nausea, vomiting, muscle cramps, or itching. By April 2000 serum creatinine level was 8.6 mg per dl. She had been advised to start dialysis but wanted to defer it because she "didn't feel that badly." Current medications included Cardizem, Lasix, Zestril, clonidine, and Claritin.

Physical exam was normal (blood pressure was 124/76, reflecting her antihypertensive drug regimen). Laboratory data showed severe kidney failure: serum creatinine 8.9 mg per dl, serum urea nitrogen 92 mg per dl, hematocrit 31 percent, serum potassium 5.6 mEq per liter, serum CO_2 19 mM. Creatinine clearance after cimetidine was 6.9, 5.7, and 5.6 ml per minute (average is 6.1 ml per minute; normal is 120 ml per minute). She was instructed on a very-low-protein diet, told where to get essential amino acids, given a prescription for a multivitamin preparation, told to take 30 grains of sodium bicarbonate daily, and sent home. Because of her employment in a clinical laboratory, she is able to conduct her own creatinine clearances after cimetidine and send me the results. She has not returned to Johns Hopkins, but we converse every two months or so and discuss her latest results. Kidney function has improved (GFR now 14 ml per minute), serum creatinine 6 mg per dl, serum urea nitrogen 68 mg per dl. Her serum CO_2 came up to normal (now 22 mM) on continued sodium bicarbonate, and her serum potassium fell to normal (now 4.9 mEq per liter) after the addition of one tablespoon per day of sodium polystyrene sulfonate. (Two tablespoonfuls a day were too much; serum potassium fell to the lower limit of normal.) Blood pressure is well regulated. Her hematocrit is 30 percent. She continues to work full time and has no symptoms. Her mild fatigue was probably attributable to her mild anemia; her health insurance has finally agreed to pay for erythropoietin treatment. She has not progressed in two and a half years. She may continue this way for years to come.

—Dialysis deferral: 4 years

Norton Cox, a 77-year-old retired NASA engineer, was referred in April 2000 with a five-year history of high blood pressure and chronic kidney failure. He also had an enlarged prostate. Despite treatment with an ACE inhibitor, serum creatinine concentration had increased to 3.3 mg per dl. He had had one episode of amnesia three years ago, which left him with some problems with memory ever since. He complained of muscle cramps, but only after playing tennis. He had no other symptoms. He was placed on a very-low-protein diet supplemented by essential amino acids. In the ensuing two years, his kidney function (measured every three months) has not changed. He remains essentially free of symptoms. He may never go on dialysis.

—Dialysis deferral: 4 years so far

Patients with Diseases of the Glomeruli

Cary Moulin, a 40-year-old laboratory technician, was referred for treatment of glomerulonephritis, known to be progressive for the previous 19 years. He was an avid jogger, running about 48 miles a week. Physical exam showed only high blood pressure. His serum creatinine level was quite high (5.5 mg per dl), as was his serum urea nitrogen level (95 mg per dl; normal is less than 22 mg per dl); yet he had few symptoms. In response to a very low-protein diet supplemented by essential amino acids, serum urea nitrogen fell to 33 mg per dl. He also received antihypertensive drugs. He alternately took supplements of either essential amino acids or ketoacids for the next five years, at which point he finally went on dialysis. Subsequently he received a transplant.

—Dialysis deferral: 5 years

Denton Farris, a former businessman, developed urinary protein and red cells at age 65. Blood tests showed that he had a kind of kidney disease called IgA nephropathy but only mild loss of kidney function. Because of recurrent muscle pains caused by a rare disorder called polymyalgia, he was taking 5 mg per day of prednisone. An ACE inhibitor was prescribed for hypertension, which necessitated the addition of sodium polystyrene sulfonate to prevent high blood potassium concentration. As his renal function declined, a very-low-protein diet was added, supplemented alternately by amino acids or ketoacids. Later, additional antihypertensive drugs and diuretics were also added. He took ketoconazole intermittently, with uncertain effects on progression. Erythropoietin injections were added. Finally, at age 74, he went on dialysis and died a year later, after withdrawing from dialysis.

—Dialysis deferral: 3 years

John Traylor, an unemployed black youth aged 23, was referred with a history of kidney disease starting at age 14, with the appearance of protein in the urine on a routine exam. A kidney biopsy showed glomerulonephritis. By age 18, serum creatinine began to rise, reaching 4.0 mg per dl.

Except for intermittent gout and high blood pressure, he had had no symptoms. Physical exam showed only obesity. (By this time blood pressure was controlled with drugs.) Blood potassium level was alarmingly high until an ACE inhibitor was discontinued. Blood pressure was hard to control. Allopurinol was prescribed for gout, but repeated episodes occurred despite the drug. A very-low-protein diet plus essential amino acids was prescribed at age 24. Kidney function continued to decline. Ketoconazole plus low-dose prednisone was added at age 27. Progression slowed. This regimen was continued for three more years, until he finally went on dialysis at age 30.

—Dialysis deferral: 4 years

Jerry Strong, a 35-year-old social worker, had developed glomerulonephritis at age 19 and had had recurrent ankle swelling and occasional gout ever since. After one year of observation, he was started on a very-low-protein diet supplemented by either essential amino acids or ketoacids. By age 39 it was clear that his kidney disease was still progressing, and ketoconazole plus low-dose prednisone was added. For the next four years he continued this regimen. During this time he complained only of muscle cramps and mild fatigue. Injections of ery-thropoietin did not help his anemia. At age 43 he received a kidney transplant from his sister.

—Dialysis deferral: 4 years

Charles Hollins, a 49-year-old hazardous waste engineer, gave a 18-year history of hypertension, with protein in the urine for at least eight years. Kidney function began to decline three years ago. A kidney biopsy showed IgA nephropathy. Gout had been a major problem, and had been treated with kidney-damaging drugs, including Indocin, but never with allopurinol. Physical exam showed high blood pressure (200/90) and ankle swelling. Kidney function was about 15 percent of normal. There was substantial loss of protein in the urine. Blood uric acid level was quite high (11.1 mg per dl). He was prescribed a very-low-protein diet, essential amino acids, sodium bicarbonate, calcium carbonate, furosemide, allopurinol, and colchicine. After a few months ketocona-zole and prednisone were added. By this time his doctors in Texas were urging him to start dialysis, but he declined. Subsequently they refused to see him in person but would sign prescriptions for him. Finally, at age 54, he succumbed to dialysis.

—Dialysis deferral: 2 years

Recipes

Vegetable Chili
⅓ cup canned low-salt mushrooms
6 fluid ounces low-salt tomato sauce
½ cup frozen sliced carrots
½ cup frozen green beans
½ cup salsa
1 teaspoon Tabasco sauce

Mix all ingredients, cover. Microwave for 4 to 5 minutes or until veg-etables are tender.
Yield: 1 serving

Nutrition information:

Calories:	150
Protein:	6.55 g
Sodium:	980 mg
Potassium:	167 mg

Quick-Mix Cake

From Virginia Schuett, *Low-Protein Cookery* (Milwaukee: University of Wisconsin Press, 1997).

1 box Duncan Hines Yellow Cake Mix®

1¼ cup water

⅓ cup canola oil

1 medium egg

Preheat oven to 350°. Prepare cake mix as directed. Pour batter into a 13 × 9 inch baking pan. Bake for 35 minutes. Cool for 5 minutes. Cut into 10 equal servings. Ice with 1 tablespoon of chocolate icing.

Yield: 10 servings

Nutrition information:

Calories:	2,920 mg per recipe; 292 mg per serving
Protein:	26.5 g per recipe; 2.65 g per serving
Sodium:	3,656 mg per recipe; 366 mg per serving
Potassium:	1,400 g per recipe; 140 g per serving

Eggplant and Red Pepper Spread

1 large eggplant (250 g)

1 small red pepper (40 g)

1 tablespoon olive oil

1 clove garlic, peeled and chopped

¼ cup chopped red pepper

1 tablespoon tomato sauce

1 tablespoon finely chopped jalapeño pepper (optional)

⅛ teaspoon salt

Wash eggplant and prick all over with a fork. Roast in the broiler for 30 minutes, rotating from time to time, until the skin is charred.

Roast the red pepper in the broiler. Peel the skin when the pepper is cooled.

Heat olive oil in a frying pan, and sauté the chopped onion and garlic.

Combine the onion, garlic, and roasted eggplant, red pepper, tomato sauce, jalapeño pepper, and salt in a blender.

Blend together until everything is processed into a smooth mixture. Serve with toasted low-protein bread.

Yield: 15 servings

Nutrition information:

Calories:	208 per recipe; 21 per serving
Protein:	2.85 g per recipe; 0.29 g per serving
Sodium:	396 mg per recipe; 40 mg per serving
Potassium:	74 mg per recipe; 7.4 mg per serving

Low-Protein Pumpkin Pie

Submitted by Martha Newswanger, *Maple Syrup Urine Disease Newsletter* 18, no. 2.

Pie Crust

¼ cup shortening

1¼ cup wheat starch

3 tablespoons applesauce

2 tablespoons corn syrup

2–2½ tablespoons water

Cut shortening into wheat starch until crumbly. Add remaining ingredients, using more wheat starch as necessary. Roll out quickly. Make a 9-inch pie crust. Set aside.

Pie Filling

¼ cup melted butter

1 cup canned pumpkin

½ cup sugar

1 cup water

2 tablespoons Ener-G Foods Egg Replacer®

2 tablespoons cornstarch

¼ cup powdered coffee creamer

Combine all ingredients in a blender in order listed. Pour into the unbaked low-protein pie shell. Sprinkle with pumpkin pie seasoning or cinnamon. Bake at 350 degrees for 45 minutes.

Yield: 8 servings

Nutrition information:

Calories:	166 per recipe; 21 per serving
Protein:	279 g per recipe; 35 g per serving
Sodium:	3,440 mg per recipe; 430 mg per serving
Potassium:	6.75 mg per recipe; 0.85 mg per serving

Cranberry and Pineapple Relish

8 ounces canned crushed pineapple

2 cups fresh or frozen cranberry, chopped

6 tablespoons sugar

2 teaspoons chopped mint

Mix all ingredients and keep refrigerated.

For diabetics: Reduce sugar to 1 tablespoon and use Splenda as a sweetener.

Yield: 10 servings, approximately 2 ounces each.

Nutrition information:

Calories:	5 per recipe; 0.5 per serving
Protein:	36 g per recipe; 3.6 g per serving
Sodium:	547 mg per recipe; 55 mg per serving
Potassium:	1.9 mg per recipe; 0.2 mg per serving

Appendix 1

Resources for Patients with Kidney Disease

BOOKS CONTAINING FOOD COMPOSITION TABLES

The following books contain tables listing the caloric, protein, and phosphorus content of various foods (but not the ratio of protein to calories nor the ratio of phosphorus to calories, listed in Chapter 7).

Blonz, ER, ed. *The Nutrition Doctor's A-to-Z Food Counter*. New York: Signet 1999.

Hamilton, E. M. N., E. N. Whitney, and F. S. Sizer. *Nutrition: Concepts and Controversies*, 3rd ed. St. Paul, MN: West Publishing Co., 1985.

Morrill, J.S., S. Bakun, and S. P. Murphy. *Are You Eating Right?: Analyze Your Diet Using the Nutrient Content of More Than 5,000 Foods*. Orange Grove Publishing, 1997.

Natow, A. B., and J. A. Heslin, *The Most Complete Food Counter*. New York: Pocket Books, 1999.

Paul, A. A., and D. A. T. Southgate. *The Composition of Foods*, 4th ed. Amsterdam: Elsevier-North Holland, 1978.

Pennington, J. A. T., A. De Planter Bowes, and H. N. Church. *Bowes & Church's Food Values of Portions Commonly Used*. Philadelphia: Lippincott Williams & Wilkins, 1998.

Sonberg, L. *The Complete Nutrition Counter*. New York: Berkeley Publishing Group, 1993.

Walser, M, A. L. Imbembo, S. Margolis, and G. A. Elfert. *Nutritional Management. The Johns Hopkins Handbook*. Philadelphia: W. B. Saunders, 1984.

Watt, B. K. *Handbook of the Nutritional Value of Foods in Common Units.* New York: Dover Publications, 1986.

INFORMATIVE BOOKS FOR PATIENTS AND THEIR PHYSICIANS

These books will supplement your reading on kidney failure and related subjects. Most of the books are primarily for dialysis patients; the exceptions are starred; some are out of print but can be obtained from your local library.

*Ahlstrom, T. P. *The Kidney Patient's Book.* Delran, N. J.: Great Issues Press, 1991.

American Association of Kidney Patients. *Patient Plan,* 2000.

Cameron, J. S. *Kidney Failure: The Facts.* New York: Oxford University Press, 1996.

Cleveland Clinic Foundation Staff. *Creative Cooking for Renal Diets.* Cleveland: Senay Publishing, 1987.

Curtis, J. A. and Batis, T. *The Renal Patient's Guide to Good Eating: A Cookbook for Patients by a Patient.* Springfield, IL: Charles C. Thomas, 2003.

*Giovannetti, S. (ed). *Nutritional Treatment of Chronic Renal Failure.* Boston: Kluwer Academic Publishers, 1989.

Hollingsworth, A. K. *Kidney Failure: Coping & Feeling Your Best.* Atlanta, GA: Pritchett & Hull Associates, 1994.

Kidney Foundation of Canada, *Living with Kidney Disease (Patient Manual),* 3rd ed. Toronto: 1999.

*Levine, D. Z. (ed). *Care of the Renal Patient.* Philadelphia: W. B. Saunders, 1991.

National Kidney and Urologic Diseases Information Clearinghouse. *Prevent Diabetes Problems: Keep Your Kidneys Healthy,* 2000.

Phillips, R. H. *Coping with Kidney Failure.* New York: Avery Publishing Group, 1987.

Schwab, S., D. W. Bartholomay, and C. W. Bales. *Eating Well, Living Well with Kidney Disease.* New York: Penguin USA, 1997.

*Schuett, V. E., *Low Protein Cookery for PKU,* 3rd ed. Milwaukee: University of Wisconsin Press, 1997.

*Vennegoor, M. (ed.). *Nutrition for Patients with Renal Failure.* London: European Dialysis and Transplant Nurses Association, European Renal Care Association, 1986.

WEB SITES

Here is a list of web sites you may find useful:

a. General Information
betterhealth.vic.gov.au
calwoodnutritionals.com
chid.nih.gov
diabeticgourmet.com
kidney.ca
nephron.com
niddk.nih.gov
onhealth.webmd.com

b. Low-Protein Web Sites and Phone Numbers
cambrookefoods.com, 508-601-1640
dietspec.com, 888-MENU123
ener-g.com, 800-331-5222
www.med-diet.com, 800-633-5550
www.shsna.com, 888-LOPROGO

USEFUL PRODUCTS FOR PATIENTS WITH KIDNEY FAILURE

Supplementation with essential amino acids (a mixture of histidine 6.25 percent, isoleucine 8.33 percent, leucine 12.5 percent, lysine acetate corresponding to lysine 9.03 percent, methionine 12.5 percent, phenylalanine 9.72 percent, threonine 9.03 percent, tryptophan 3.47 percent, tyrosine 10.42 percent, valine 18.75 percent) is vital to anyone on a very-low-protein diet.

Powder and Candies

Nutramine contains the above-listed amino acids, 3.5 g per serving, plus additives to mask taste. Available from Calwood Nutritionals, Inc., 500 McCormick Drive, Suite J, Glen Burnie, MD 21061; calwoodnutritionals.com; 800-479-9942. Dose: 3 servings per day with meals.

Tablets

Aminess N contains 720 mg of the listed amino acids per tablet. Distributed by Gambro Renal Products Inc., Lakewood, CA 80215, www.usa-gambro.com; 303-239-2188. Dose: 15 tablets per day, taken with meals. (The dose is incorrectly stated on the label.)

Other mixtures of amino acids that are on the market do not contain these same amino acids and are less effective.

Drugs Available without a Prescription

Sodium bicarbonate: 10 grain (650 mg) tablets
Cimetidine (Tagamet®): 200 mg or 300 mg tablets
Tums®: 400 mg calcium carbonate

Diagnostic Agents

Paper test strips for protein and glucose in the urine
Paper test strips for pH, protein, ketones, urobilinogen, bilirubin, glucose, nitrite, blood, and white blood cells in the urine
To order more of these test strips, call 800-443-9942

Prescription Drugs Used Particularly in Kidney Failure

Disalcid: Salsalate (salicyl salicylate). Dose: 1 to 3 g per day.
Procrit and Epogen: Identical formulations of erythropoietin alpha for injection (see Chapter 11), produced by recombinant DNA technology. Dose: 50 to 100 units per kg, three times a week, intravenously or subcutaneously.
Iron sucrose (iron saccharate): Weekly Dose: 100 mg intravenously, (see Chapter 11).
Kionex: Sodium polystyrene sulfonate, an ion exchange resin that is not absorbed from the gut, but takes up potassium in exchange for sodium and is excreted in the stool. (See Chapter 12.) Dose: 15 to 60 g per day, to be taken in three divided doses in syrup by mouth, with a laxative if needed, or, if necessary, by enema.
Nephrocaps and Nephrovites: Almost identical formulations containing all of the water-soluble vitamins but omitting the fat-soluble vitamins. Dose: 1 per day.
Rocaltrol capsules: Calcitriol (the active form of vitamin D; see Chapter 13). Dose: 0.25 micrograms per day.

Appendix 2

Government Support of Low-Protein Diets

You may wonder why, if dietary treatment is so helpful, and if the government is expending enormous sums for the care of kidney patients, the government has not tried to expand the use of dietary treatment. It would seem that huge savings as well as improved care could result. The answer is rather complex, but may be worth your examining in detail. Public pressure is what gets such studies funded in the first place. Because government support for research on dietary treatment has so far led to disappointing or equivocal results, government interest is minimal. The proper response should be to do better studies, rather than to give up. You can help by writing your congressman and urging additional funding for studies of how to slow the progression of kidney disease.

Many years ago two small studies on the effects on progression of patients on a very-low-protein diet supplemented with ketoacids were published. Both provided evidence of substantial slowing of progression in both diabetic and nondiabetic renal disease. The same diet supplemented by essential amino acids instead of ketoacids appeared to be less effective in this regard, although some evidence of rather poor quality pointed to slowing by this regimen too. A low-protein diet (40 to 60 g per day) without a supplement has been the subject of many studies, some better controlled than others, with mixed results.

In the 1970s, two colleagues from industry and I lobbied Congress and eventually persuaded members that the government should test the hypothesis that protein-controlled products could slow the progression of renal failure toward the end stage. We based our information on my own data and data from Giuseppe Maschio from Italy. Two legislators who were particularly helpful were Al Gore and

Bob Dole. The law Congress passed instructed the secretary of Health, Education, and Welfare to conduct such a study and to report to Congress. This "mandate" went over like a lead balloon at the National Institutes of Health (NIH), which hates to be told what to do. Also, many academic nephrologists were justly concerned that an expensive project such as this could divert research funds away from other more basic projects, many of which were in fact their main research efforts. Fifteen nephrologists and I wrote to Richard M. Schweiker, secretary of Health and Human Services, on May 17, 1982, urging the government to conduct a study of the effects of dietary treatment upon the progression, symptoms, and clinical course of renal failure.

We also strongly urged that these funds not be taken from the NIH funds presently allocated to kidney research, funds that were barely adequate and might be significantly depleted by the costs of the study.

About this time NIH and HCFA (the Health Care Financing Administration, which administers the Medicaid and Medicare programs) decided to move forward. They assembled a steering committee, including me, to meet for a year to plan the study. I was specifically instructed to say nothing when the question of whether to include ketoacids was discussed, because the ketoacid patents had been assigned to my employer, Johns Hopkins University, and this produced the appearance of a conflict of interest. Nevertheless the group decided to include the ketoacid-supplemented very-low-protein diet as one arm of the study. In the Feasibility Phase of the study, which was not intended to establish the efficacy of any regimen but rather to uncover any possible problems, another group of patients was to receive a very-low-protein diet supplemented with essential amino acids. It was agreed that a normal-protein diet was not an ethical alternative for patients with advanced renal failure, since such a regimen would probably increase their symptoms. Consequently, the study had to be divided into two separate studies: one in early renal failure, in which a normal protein-containing diet was one arm; and a second in more advanced renal failure, in which a low-protein diet was compared to a supplemented very-low-protein diet. No attempt was made to regulate blood pressure to any particular level. Insulin-dependent diabetic patients were excluded, because the problems of achieving good diabetic control with different diets seemed an insurmountable extra burden. It was agreed that renal function would be measured four times a year by the radioisotope technique, collecting three urine samples and averaging the three clearance periods.

The Feasibility Phase enrolled only 30 patients in Study A (with less severe renal failure) and only 66 in Study B (with more severe renal failure). To be enrolled in the study, each patient's previous serum creatinine values had to give evidence of progression of their disease. This was a crucial point, as I will explain later.

Patients were to be followed for two years. In fact, average follow-up was only 14 months. Compliance to the diet was rather poor. Initial reports stated that there was no difference in progression rates between the different diet groups. This statement was later retracted, and a significant slowing of progression in the ketoacid-supplemented group as compared with the essential amino acid–supplemented group was documented. This was a surprise, as we believed the Feasibility Phase was far too small to establish the superiority of one treatment over another.

The explanation of the erroneous initial reports remains unknown, but the release of this information at the end of the Feasibility Phase could have jeopardized the continuance of the study into the Operational Phase, for ethical reasons.

In the Feasibility Phase, the ketoacid mixture employed was the one called EE, designed and patented at Johns Hopkins and manufactured in France. It was by design devoid of tryptophan, for various reasons. The Steering Committee met at the end of the Feasibility Phase and decided to make one change in the ketoacid mixture to be used in the Operational Phase (the main study): A small amount of tryptophan was to be added. Later we reported our findings that patients' serum free tryptophan levels often fell progressively on EE , so in retrospect this addition seemed a rational decision. No other changes in the ketoacid mixture were ordered.

Nevertheless, Ross Laboratories, the source selected (instead of the French company) to supply EE, without authorization or notification, made a number of other changes. Instead of EE, during the Operational Phase Ross Laboratiories supplied its own patented ketoacid mixture, a very different formulation. No one recognized this switch because of the complex formulation that appeared on the label. The study went forward without anyone (except Ross Laboratories) knowing what was being studied. This may be a unique example of a huge clinical trial funded by the government at over $100 million in which neither the government nor the investigators knew what they were studying.

Another striking feature of the Feasibility Phase results was the strong dependence of progression rate on blood pressure. Because of the design of the study, it could not be determined whether high levels of blood pressure caused faster progression or whether patients with rapidly progressing renal disease also tend to have higher blood pressures. So a second major change in the protocol was introduced for the next phase: Patients were to be assigned by chance to two different blood pressure targets. Also, the requirement that patients' prior creatinine measurements give evidence of progression was dropped for statistical reasons. This was a major error, to my way of thinking. In the end, 15 percent of the patients studied were not progressing even before the study started. This is like trying to determine the efficacy of a drug for tuberculosis in a group of patients that includes 15 percent who don't have tuberculosis. The essential amino acid arm was also dropped. It was determined that I had the appearance of a conflict of interest, being on the Johns Hopkins faculty, and I was asked to withdraw.

When the results of the Operational Phase were published in 1994, skeptics seized on the primary analysis, which showed only marginally significant differences in progression rates between the diet groups, and concluded that diet had no place in the treatment of renal failure.

This conclusion was premature. More detailed analysis showed that, after the initial decline in glomerular filtration rate caused by the reduction in protein intake, patients on the supplemented very-low-protein diet progressed more slowly than those on the 40 g protein diet. This difference persisted until the end of the study at two years; if this difference in progression rates had continued for five years, the difference in final glomerular filtration rate and in the fraction of patients who reached end-stage renal disease would have been considerable. Secondary analyses, using the measurements of 24-hour urine urea nitrogen excretion to estimate actual protein intake, supported the view that protein restriction had indeed slowed progression.

The costs of the study far exceeded initial predictions: nearly $100 million was spent, with both HCFA and NIH paying a portion.

Despite this enormous expenditure, the study failed in many ways. It failed to settle the question as to whether any degree of protein restriction slows disease progression. Three groups of authors have applied meta-analysis to this question. They have assembled published reports and showed the mean effect on progression (compared to controls) of protein restriction in each, as well as the confidence limits of the difference. (Confidence limits mean the possible upper and lower limits of the range of values for the quantity being estimated, within the limits of probability.) These data, plotted together on a single graph, give a good picture of the range of findings and may lead to a conclusion from apparently contradictory data. A major problem with meta-analysis is deciding which studies to include, and nowhere is this problem shown more dramatically than in a comparison of these three published meta-analyses of progression on protein-restricted diets. Each has selected different publications to include, and each has reached slightly different conclusions. But the general impression these reports give is that protein restriction does slow progression.

Recently Andrew Levey and his colleagues have summarized all of these Modification of Diet in Renal Disease results, concluding "the balance of evidence is more consistent with the hypothesis of beneficial effect of protein restriction [on progression of renal failure] than with the contrary hypothesis of no beneficial effect" and "a very low protein diet supplemented with a mixture of ketoacids and amino acids may also be beneficial, but differences in study design and in the composition of the supplements make it difficult to determine whether the very low protein diets are more beneficial than a low protein diet."

Notes

p. 2: *"At least 6 million people…"*: C. A. Jones, G. M. McQuillan, J .W. Kusek, M. S. Everhardt, W. H. Herman, J. Coresh, M. Salive, C. P. Jones, and L. Y. Agoda, "Serum Creatinine Levels in the U. S. Population: Third National Health and Nutrition Examination Survey," *American Journal of Kidney Diseases* 32 (1998): 992–999.

p. 2: *Official government report of the U. S. Renal Data System:* U. S. Renal Data System (USRDS), 1999, 2000, and 2001 Annual Data Reports, National Institutes of Health.

p. 2: *a "good death":* L. M. Cohen, M. J. Germain, D. M. Poppel, A. L. Woods, and C. M. Kjellstarnd, "Dying Well after Discontinuing Life-Support Treatment of Dialysis," *Archives of Internal Medicine* 160 (2000): 2513–2518.

p. 13: *Prevalence of …kidney disease in the United States:* A. X. Garg, B. A. Kiberd, W. F. Clark, R. B. Haynes, and C. M. Clase, "Albuminuria and Renal Insufficiency Prevalence Guides Population Screening: Results from the NHANES III," *Kidney International* 61 (2002): 2165–2175.

p. 13: "Do all patients progress?: J. C. Fink, M Salmanullah, S. A. Blahut, M. R. Weir, R. Sawyer, W. L. Henrich, and M. K. Hise, "The Inevitability of Renal Function Loss in Patients with Hypercreatininemia," *American Journal of Nephrology* 21 (2001): 386–389. S. Rottey, R. Vanholder, G. DeSchoenmakere, and N. Lemeire, "Progression of Renal Failure in Patients with Compromised Renal Function Is Not Always Present: Evaluation of Underlying Disease," *Clinical Nephrology* 54 (2000): 1–10.

p. 14: Progressors and nonprogressors in the MDRD study: A. S. Levey, T. Greene, G. J. Beck, A. W. Caggiula, J. W. Kusek, L. G. Hunsicker, and S. Klahr, "Dietary Protein Restriction and the Progression of Chronic Renal Disease: What Have All of the Results of the MDRD Study Show?" *Journal of the American Society of Nephrology* 10 (1999): 2426–2439.

p. 14: *A survey of 1,436 adults in Venezuela:* F. Aguero, P. I. Santacruz, D. Urbina, O. Zarraga, and C. Aguero, "Prevalence of Chronic Renal Failure (CRF) in a General Population: An Epidemiological Approach," *Nephrology Dialysis Transplantation* 16 (2001): A105.

p.14: *In a survey of 23,121 healthy Japanese schoolchildren:* M. J. Pugia, M. Murakami, Y. Ohta, T. Kitagawa, K. Ymamuchi, Y. Suhara, and J. Kasjima, "Screening for Proteinuria in Japanese Schoolchildren: A New Approach," *Clinical Chemistry and Laboratory Medicine* 38 (2000): 975–982.

p. 14: *In a large survey:* See Jones et a., "Serum Creatinine Levels."

p. 15: *Difference between true prevalence and diagnosed disease:* W. M. McClellan, D. F.

Knight, H. Karp, and W. W. Brown, "Early Detection and Treatment of Renal Disease in Hospitalized Diabetic and Hypertensive Patients: Important Differences between Practice and Published Guidelines," *American Journal of Kidney Diseases* 29 (1997): 368–375.

p. 15: *Diabetic Medicare beneficiaries…from Seattle:* "ACE Inhibitors in the Treatment of Diabetic Nephropathy in Washington," Report by PRO-West, Seattle, Washington, 1995, 1–16.

p. 15: *Recent report by Italian nephrologists:* C. Catalano, V. Brodin, G. Panebianco, D. Lambertini, F. Fabbian, D. Di Landro, "Identification of Renal Damage and of Risk Markers for Renal Damage in a Cohort of Diabetic Outpatients," *Nephrology Dialysis Transplantation* 14 (1999): 248.

p. 16: *"An alarmingly poor quality of pre-ERSD care…":* G. T. Obrador, P. Arora, A. T. Kausz, S. S. Khan, R. Abichandani, W. H. Kazmi, G. T. Obrador, R. Ruthazer, and B. J. G. Pereira, "Management of Patients with Chronic Renal Insufficiency in the Northeastern United States," *Journal of the American Society of Nephrology* 12 (2001): 1501–1507.

p. 16: *Recent pamphlet for the general public:* National Institute of Diabetes and Digestive and Kidney Diseases, "Kidney Failure: Choosing a Treatment That's Right for You." NIH Publication No. 01-2412, 2001.

p. 18: The prevalence of kidney disease among relatives of dialysis patients: D. A. Molony, personal communication, 2000. D. A. Molony, W. W. Brown, K. King, and M. Gannon, "Screening of High-Risk Populations Identifies a High Prevalence of Individuals with Abnormal Renal Function: the NKF Early Evaluation Program," *Journal of the American Society of Nephrology* 11, (2000): 158A.

p. 19: Urinary protein as a predictor of kidney failure in people with diabetes: M. L. Caramori, P Fioretto, and M. Mauer, "The Need for Early Predictors of Diabetic Nephropathy Risk," *Diabetes* 49, (2000): 1399–1408.

p. 20: *Controlling blood pressure in nonmalignant hypertension…doesn't make any difference:* C. Y. Hsu, "Does Treatment of Non-Malignant Hypertension Reduce the Incidence of Renal Dysfunction? A Meta-Analysis of 10 Randomised, Controlled Trials," *Journal of Human Hypertension* 15 (2001): 99-106.

p. 20: Hypertension as a cause of kidney failure: N. M. Kaplan and E. Lieberman, *Kaplan's Clinical Hypertension*, 8th ed. (Philadelphia: Lippincott Williams & Wilkins, 2002).

p. 21: *Potassium deficiency is another cause of kidney failure:* A. S. Relman and W. B. Schwartz, "The Nephropathy of Potassium Depletion," *New England Journal of Medicine* 255 (1956): 195–203.

p. 22: Kidney disease caused by analgesics: R. E. Cronin and W. L. Henrich, "Toxic Nephropathies," in *The Kidney*, 6th ed., B. M. Brenner (Philadelphia: W. B. Saunders, 2000), 1563–1596. T. V. Perneger, P. K. Whelton, and M. J. Klag, "Risk of Kidney Failure Associated with the Use of Acetaminophen, Aspirin, and Nonsteroidal Anti-Inflammatory Drugs," *New England Journal of Medicine* 331 (1994): 1675–1679.

p. 25: *Evidence supporting the idea that high protein intake damages the kidney is unconvincing:* D. C. Tapp, W. G. Wortham, F. J. Addison, D. N. Hammonds, J. L. Barnes, and M. A. Venkatachalam, "Food Restriction Retards Body Growth and

Prevents End-Stage Renal Pathology in Remnant Kidney of Rats Regardless of Protein Intake," *Laboratory Investigation* 60 (1989): 184–195.

p. 25: High protein intake doesn't cause kidney insufficiency in normal rats: D. M. Collins, C. T. Rezzo, J. B. Kopp, P. Ruiz, D. M. Coffman, and P. E. Klotman, "Chronic High Protein Feeding Does Not Produce Glomerulosclerosis or Renal Insufficiency in the Normal Rat" [abstract], *Journal of the American Society of Nephrology*10 (1999): 81A.

p. 25: *Doubt on the idea that protein harms normal kidneys:* S. Q. Lew and J. P. Bosch, "Effects of Diet on Creatinine Clearance and Excretion in Young and Elderly Healthy Subjects and in Patients in Renal Disease," *Journal of the American Society of Nephrology* 2 (1992): 856–865.

p. 26: *Other species do not exhibit the progressive decline in kidney function:* J. J. Bourgoignie, G. Gavellas, S. G. Sabnis, and T. T. Antonovych, "Effect of Protein Diets on the Renal Function of Baboons (*Papio hamadryas*) with Remnant Kidneys. A 5-Year Follow-up," *American Journal of Kidney Diseases* 23 (1994): 199–204. K. C. Bovée, "High Dietary Protein Intake Does Not Cause Progressive Renal Failure in Dogs after 75% Nephrectomy or Aging," *Seminars in Veterinary Medical Surgery (Small Animals)* 7 (1992): 227–236. K. C. Bovée, "Influence of Dietary Protein on Renal Function in Dogs," *Journal of Nutrition* 121 (Suppl.) (1991): S128–S139.

p. 30: *A life-threatening bleeding disorder:* J. R. Brasic, "Quinine-induced Thrombocytopenia in a 64-Year-Old Man Who Consumed Tonic Water to Relieve Nocturnal Leg Cramps," *Mayo Clinic Proceedings* 76 (2001): 863–864.

p. 31: *Symptoms...the consequence of chemical abnormalities:* R. Mazhari and M. Walser, "Dependence of the Symptoms of Chronic Renal Disease on Biochemical Changes," *Journal of the American Society of Nephrology* [abstract] 10 (1999): 81A.

p. 32: *Nausea and vomiting...correlated with the concentration of albumin in the serum:* B. Klang, H. Björvell, and N. Clyne, "Quality of Life in Predialytic Uremic Patients," *Quality of Life Research* 5 (1996) 109–116. B. Klang and N. Clyne, "Well-being and Functional Ability in Uremic Patients Before and After Having Started Dialysis Treatment." *Scandinavian Journal of Caring Science* 11 (1997): 159–166.

p. 35: *To quote Dr. Robert Berliner:* Berliner, R. W. Foreword in: *The Kidney*, edited by B. M. Brenner, Rector F. C. Philadelphia: Saunders, 1976, pp. xii.

p. 36: *Experience with an artificial kidney in dogs:* J. J. Abel, L. G. Rowntree, and B. B. Turner, "On the Removal of Diffusible Substances from the Circulating Blood of Living Animal by Dialysis," *Journal of Pharmacology and Experimental Therapeutics* 5 (1913–1914): 275.

p. 36: *A Dutch physician...and his associates first successfully used an artificial kidney:* W. J. Kolff, H. T. Berk, M. ter Welle, A. J. van der Ley, E. C. van Dijk, and J. Noordwijk, "Artificial Kidney: A Dialyzer with Great Area," *Acta Medica Scandinavica* 117 (1944): 121–134. Reprinted in *Journal of the American Society of Nephrology* 8 (1997): 1959–1965. B. H. Scribner, R. S. Biri, J. E. Z. Caner, R. Hegstrom, and J. M. Burnell, "The Treatment of Uremia by Means of Intermittent Dialysis: A Preliminary Report," *Transactions of the American Society of Artificial Internal Organs* 6 (1960): 114–117.

p. 38: *Withdrawal from dialysis is...a "good death":* Cohen, L. M., Germain, M. J., Poppel, D. M., Woods, A. L., and Kjellstrand, C. M., "Dying Well after

Discontinuing the Life-Support Treatment of Dialysis." *Archives of Internal Medicine* 160 (2000): 2513–2518.

p. 40: *At least one-third of these patients have succeeded in deferring dialysis:* M. Walser and S. Hill, "Can Renal Replacement Be Deferred by a Supplemented Very-Low-Protein Diet?" *Journal of the American Society of Nephrology* 10 (1999): 110–116. M. Aparicio, P. Chauveau, V. De Précigout, J.-L. Bouchet, C. Lasseur, and C. Combe, "Nutrition and Outcome in Renal Replacement Therapy of Patients with Chronic Renal Failure Treated by a Supplemented Very-Low-Protein Diet," *Journal of the American Society of Nephrology* 11, (2000): 708–716.

p. 40: *Interval between diagnosis of renal failure and the start of dialysis:* M. Walser, V. Stallings, and T. Hutchinson, "Characterization of Progression of Chronic Renal Failure," *Clinical Research* [abstract] 32 (1984): 565A.

p. 41: *Other nephrologists have become increasingly skeptical:* G. Schulman, and R, M. Hakim, "Improving Outcomes in Chronic Hemodialysis Patients: Should Dialysis Be Started Earlier?" *Seminars in Dialysis* 9 (1996): 225–229.

p. 41: *A protein-restricted diet before being placed on dialysis:* M. Walser, W. E. Mitch, B. J. Maroni, and J. D. Kopple, "Should Protein Intake Be Restricted in Pre-Dialysis Patients?" *Kidney International* 55 (1999): 771–777.

p. 53: *Smoking hastens the progression of kidney disease:* T. Chuahirun, A. Khanna, K. Kimball, and D. E. Wesson, "Cigarette Smoking and Increased Albumin Excretion Are Interrelated Predictors of Nephropathy Progression in Type 2 Diabetes," *American Journal of Kidney Diseases* 41 (2003): 13–21. M. Tozaa, K. Ideki, C. Iseki, S. Oshiro, Y., Ikemiya, and S. Takashita, "Influence of Smoking and Obesity on the Development of Proteinuria," *Kidney International* 62, (2002): 956–962. E. M. Briganti, P. Branley, S. J. Chadban, J. E. Shaw, J. J. McNeil, T. A. Welborn, and R. C. Atkins, "Smoking Is Associated with Renal Impairment and Proteinuria in the Normal Population: The Australian Diabetes, Obesity and Lifestyle Study," *Journal of Kidney Diseases* 40 (2002): 704–712.

p. 54: *No reason for people with kidney failure to avoid strenuous activity:* M. L. Boyce, R. A. Robergs, P. S. Avasthi, R. Roldan, A. Foster, P. Montner, D. Stark, and C. Nelson, " Exercise Training by Individuals with Predialysis Renal Failure: Cardiorespiratory Endurance, Hypertension, and Renal Function," *American Journal of Kidney Diseases* 30 (1997): 180–192. N. Clyne, J. Ekholm, T. Jogestrand, L.E. Linds, and S. K. Pehrsson, "Effects of Exercise Training in Predialytic Uremic Patients," *Nephron* 59 (1999): 84–89.

p. 56: *If these eight amino acids are ingested…no protein at all in the diet is needed:* W. C. Rose, "Amino Acid Requirements in Man," *Federation Proceedings* 8 (149); 546–552.

p. 57: *The low-protein diet pioneered by Franz Volhard:* F. Volhard, "Die doppelseitigen hämatogenen Neirenkrankungen (Bright'sche Krankheit)," in *Handbuch der Inneren Medizen*, (Berlin: Springer, 1918), 1149–1172, special p. 1400.

p. 57: *High-protein foods aggravate several aspects of kidney failure:* E. L. Knight, M. J. Stampfer, S. E. Hankinson, D. Spiegelman and G. C. Curhan, "The Impact of Protein Intake on Renal Function Decline in Women with Normal Renal Function or Mild Renal Insufficiency," *Annals of Internal Medicine* 18: 2003): 460–467.

p. 58: *People with kidney failure…should avoid star fruit:* H.-J. Yap, Y.-C. Chen, J. T.

Fang, C.-C. Huang, "Star Fruit: A Neglected but Serious Fruit Intoxicant in Chronic Renal Failure," *Dialysis and Transplantation* 31 (2002): 564–597.

p. 66: *A former patient of mine:* T. P. Ahlstrom, *The Kidney Patient's Book* (Delran, NJ: Great Issues Press, 1991).

p. 67: *Virginia E. Schuett has written a book:* V. E. Schuett, *Low Protein Cookery for PKU*, 3rd ed, (Milwaukee: University of Wisconsin Press, 1997).

p. 82: *First...use of very-low-protein diets supplemented by essential amino acids:* C. Giordano, "Use of Exogenous and Endogenous Urea for Protein Synthesis in Normal and Uremic Subjects," *Journal of Laboratory and Clinical Medicine* 62 (1963): 231–246. S. Giovannetti and Q. Maggiore, "A Low-Nitrogen Diet with Proteins of High Biological Value for Severe Chronic Uremia," *Lancet* 1(1964): 1000–1003.

p. 82: *This very low intake of protein is acceptable:* L.-O. Norée and J. Bergström, Treatment of Chronic Uremic Patients with Protein-Poor Diet and Oral Supply of Essential Amino Acids. II. Clinical Results of Long-Term Treatment," *Clinical Nephrology* 3 (1975): 195–2000.

p. 83: Acceptability of the Bergström diet: D. Kampf, H. C. Fischer, and M. Kessel, "Efficacy of an Unselected Protein Diet (25g) with Minor Oral Supply of Essential Amino Acids and Keto Analogues Compared with Selective Protein Diet (40g) in Chronic Renal Failure," *American Journal of Clinical Nutrition* 33 (1980): 1673–1677.

p. 83: *In a randomized nine-month study:* J. Kult, "Serum Levels of Trace Proteins in Continued Substitution of Essential Amino Acids Combined with Low Protein Diet in Patients with Endstage Renal Failure," *Renal Insufficiency* ed., A Heidland, (Stuttgart: Georg Thieme Verlag, 1976), p. 169. A Röckel, F. Roller, J. Kult, and A Heidland, "Comparative Studies of Potato-Egg Diet and Mixed Low Protein Diet Combined with Essential Amino Acid in Patients with Endstage Renal Failure." in *Renal Insufficiency*, ed. A. Heidland (Stuttgart: Georg Thieme Verlag, 1976), p. 163.

p. 85: Essential amino acids maintain protein nutrition without dietary protein: W. C. Rose, "Amino Acid Requirements in Man," *Federation Proceedings* 8 (149); 546–553.

p. 86: *Study...on 29 patients on hemodialysis:* J. A. Eustace, J. Coresh, C. Kutchey, P. L. Te, L. F. Gimenez, P. J. Scheel Jr., and M. Walser, "Randomized Double-Blind Trial of Oral Essential Amino Acids for Dialysis-Associated Hypoalbuminemia," *Kidney International* 57 (2000): 2527–2538.

p. 87: The MDRD Study, Klahr S, Levey AS, Beck GJ, et al: The effects of dietary protein restriction and blood-pressure control on the progression of chronic renal failure. *New England Journal of Medicine* 330:878–884, 1994.

p. 99: *People with diabetes and kidney disease:* G. L. Bakris, M. R. Weir, S. Sahanifar, Z. Zhang, J. Douglas, D. J. van Dijk, and B. M. Brenner, "RENAAL Study Group," *Archives of Internal Medicine* 14 (2003): 1555–1565.

p. 110: *Some authors report that progression slows with such treatment:* M. Tapolya, S. Kadomatsu, and M. Perera-Chong, "Rhu-Erythropoietin (EPO) Treatment of Pre-ESRD Patients Slows the Rate of Progression of Renal Decline," *BMC Nephrology* 17 (2003): 3.

p. 110: Iron deficiency in renal failure: A. M. Fernandez-Rodriguez, M. C. Guindeo-Casasus, T. Molero-Labarta, C. Dominquez-Cabrera, L. Hortal-Cascon, P.

Perez-Borges, N. Vega-Diaz, P. Saavedra-Santana, L. Palop-Cubillo, "Diagnosis of Iron Deficiency in Chronic Renal Failure," *American Journal of Kidney Diseases* 34 (199): 508–513.

p. 111: Intravenous iron treatment: Van Wyck, D. B. Cavallo, G., Spinowitz, B. S., Adhirkarla, R., Gagnon, S., Charytan, C., and Levin, N. "Safety and Efficacy of Iron Sucrose in Patients Sensitive to Iron Dextran: North American Clinical Trial." *American Journal of Kidney Diseases* 36 (2000): 88–97.

p. 114: *Hyperkaliemia as a result of taking an ACE inhibitor:* T. W. Ahuja, D. Freeman, J. D. Mahnken, M. Agraharkar, M. Siddiqui, and A. Memon, "Predictors of the Development of Hyperkaliemia in Patients using Angiotensin-Converting Enzyme Inhibitors," *American Journal of Nephrology* 20 (2000): 268–272.

p. 120: Low-phosphorus diet for reducing parathyroid hormone and increasing vitamin D Levels: N. Areste, J. Amor, T. Cambill, M. Salgueira, S. R. Sanchez-Palencia, C. Paez, O. Gomez, and A. Palma [Early Treatment of Secondary Hyperparathyroidism in Moderate Renal Insufficiency: Low-Phosphorus Diet versus Calcium Carbonate]. *Nephrologia* 23, Supplement 2 (2003): 64–68.

p. 120: *A simple formula gives a good estimate:* J. H. Barth, J. B. Fiddy, and R. B. Payne, "Adjustment of Serum Total Calcium for Albumin Concentration: Effects of Non-Linearity and of Regression Differences between Laboratories," *Annals of Clinical Biochemistry* 33 (1996): 55–58.

p. 121: A new phosphate binder: E. A. Slatopolsky, S. K. Burke, M. A. Dillon, and The RenaGel® Study Group, "RenaGel®, a Nonabsorbed Phosphate Binder, Lowers Serum Phosphate and Parathyroid Hormone," *Kidney International* 55 (1999): 299–307.

p. 124: *Patients...given...colchicine...who developed severe neuromyopathy:* J. J. Montseny, A. Meyrier, and R. K. Gherardi, "Colchicine Toxicity in Patients with Chronic Renal Failure," *Nephrology Dialysis Transplantation* 11 (1996): 2055–2058.

p. 125: *Occasional patient exhibit low uric acid levels:* Y. Kikiuchi, H. Koga, Y. Yasumoto, Y. Kawabata, E. Shimuzi, M. Naruse, S. Kiyama, H. Nonoguchi, K. Tomita, Y. Sasatomi, and S. Takebayashi, "Patients with Renal Hperuricemia with Exercise-Induced Acute Renal Failure and Chronic Renal Dysfunction," *Clinical Nephrology* 53 (2000): 467–472.

p. 131: Slowing of progression by ACE inhibitors: A. V. Kshiragar, M. S. Joy, S. L. Hogan, R. J. Falk, and R. E. Colindres, "Effect of ACE Inhibitors in Diatetic and Nondiabetic Chronic Renal Disease: A Systematic Overview of Randomized Placebo-Controlled Trials," *American Journal of Kidney Diseases* 35 (2000): 695–707.

p. 131: Slowing of progression by an angiotensin receptor blocker: B. M. Brenner, M. E. Cooper, D. de Zeeuw, W. F. Keane, W. E. Mitch, H.-H. Parving, G. Remuzzi, S. M. Snappin, Z. Zhang, and S. Shahinfar, "Effects of Losartan on Renal and Cardiovascular Outcomes in Patients with Type 2 Diabetes and Nephropathy," *New England Journal of Medicine* 345 (2001): 861–869.

p. 131: Late results with ACE inhibitors: T. Shiigai and M. Shichiri, "Late Escape from the Antiproteinuric Effect of ACE Inhibitors in Nondiabetic Renal Disease," *American Journal of Kidney Diseases* 37 (2001): 477–493.

p. 132: *Ketoconazole...might lead to slower progression of renal disease:* M. Walser and

S. Hill, "Effect of Ketoconazole Plus Low-dose Prednisone on Progression of Chronic Renal Failure," *American Journal of Kidney Diseases* 29 (1997): 503–513.

p. 134: *Chances of...developing clinically significant liver toxicity...with ketoconazole:* L. A. Garcia Rodriguez, A. J. Castellsague, S. Perez-Gutthann, and B. H. C. Stricker, "A Cohort Study on the Risk of Acute Liver Injury Among Users of Ketoconazole and Other Antifungal Drugs," *British Journal of Clinical Pharmacology* 48 (1999): 847–852.

p. 142: *The constant infusion technique:* A. Al-Uzri, M. A. Holliday, J. G. Gambertoglio, M. Schambelan, B. A. Kogan, and B. R. Don, "An Accurate Practical Method for Estimating GFR in Clinical Studies Using a Constant Subcutaneous Infusion," *Kidney International* 41 (1992): 1701–1706.

p. 147: *Cimetidine-modified creatinine clearance:* F. A. Kemperman, J. Surachno, R. T. Kredict, and L. Arisz, " Cimetidine Improves Prediction of the Glomerular Filtration Rate by the Cockroft-Gault Formula in Renal Transplant Recipients," *Transplantation* 73 (2002): 770–774.

p. 151: *Cystatin C...better than creatinine to determine the level of kidney function:* A. Christensson, J. Ekberg, A. Grubb, H Ekberg, V. Lindstrom, and H. Lilja, "Serum Cystatin C Is a More Sensitive and More Accurate Marker of Glomerular Filtration Rate than Enzymatic Measurements of Creatinine in Renal Transplantation," *Nephron* 94 (2003): 19–27. M. Mussap, M. Dalla Vestra, P. Fioretto, A Saller, M. Varagnolo, R. Nosadini, and M. Plebani, "Cystatin C Is a More Sensitive Marker than Creatinine for the Estimation of GFR in Type 2 Diabetic Patients," *Kidney International* 61 (2002): 1453–1461.

p. 151: Cystatin C as a GFR marker: O Schuck, V. Teplan, A, Joabor, M. Stollova, and J. Skibova, "Glomerular Filtration Rate Estimation in Patients with Advanced Chronic Renal Insufficiency Based on Serum Cystatin C Levels," *Nephron Clinical Practice* 93 (2003): 146–151.

p. 156: *Measurements from Sweden:* P. Stenvinkel, O. Heimburger, F. Paultre, U. Diczfalusy, T. Wang, L. Berglund, and T. Jogestrand, "Strong Association between Malnutrition, Inflammation, and Atherosclerosis in Chronic Renal Failure," *Kidney International* 55 (1999): 1899–1922. R. M. Hakim and J. M. Lazarus, "Biochemical Parameters in Chronic Renal Failure," *American Journal of Kidney Diseases* 11 (1988): 238–247. O. Heimburger, A. R. Qureshi Aar, W. S. Blaner, L. Berglund, and P. Stenvinkel, "Hand-Grip Strength, Lean Body Mass, and Plasma Proteins as Markers of Nutritional Status in Patients with Renal Failure Close to the Start of Dialysis Therapy," *American Journal of Kidney Disease* 36 (2000): 1213–1225.

p. 159: *In the mid-1980s:* J. van der Meulen, L. Gooren, and P. L. Oe, "Low-Protein Diet Increases Serum Albumin by Reducing Proteinuria in Some Nephrotic Patients" [abstract], *Kidney International* 28 (1985): 299.

p. 159: Treatment of the nephrotic syndrome by dietary protein restriction: M. Walser, S. Hill, and E. A. Tomalis, "Treatment of Nephrotic Adults with a Supplemented Very Low Protein Diet," *American Journal of Kidney Diseases* 28 (1996): 354–364. S. Sistani and M. Walser, "The Effect of a Supplemented Very Low Protein Diet on Proteinuria [abstract]," *Journal of the American Society of Nephrology* 11 (2000): 98A.

p. 162: *Similar results…from Japan:* T. Ideura, A. Yoshimura, and M. Shimazui, "Effect of a Very Low Protein Diet in the Nephrotic Syndrome [abstract]," *Wiener Klinische Wochenschrift* 110, Suppl. 4, 9th International Congress on Nutrition and Metabolism in Renal Disease (1997): 61.

p. 163: Drug prescribing in kidney failure: G. R. Aronoff (ed.), *Drug Prescribing in Renal Failure: Dosing Guidelines for Adults*, 4th ed. American College of Physicians (1999). A. J. Olyaei, A. M. de Mattos, and W. M. Bennett, "Prescribing Drugs in Renal Disease," in *The Kidney*, ed. B. M. Brenner (Philadelphia; W. B. Saunders, 2000).

p. 167: *Transplantation:* D. J. Dixon and S. E. Abbey, "Religious Altruism and Organ Donation," *Psychosomatics* 41 (2000): 407–411. S. C. Jacobs, E. Cho, B. J. Dunkin, J. L. Flowers, E. Schweitzer, C. Congro, J. Fink, A. Farney, B. Philosophe, B. Jarrell, and S. T. Bartlett, "Lapraroscopic Live Donor Nephrectomy: The University of Maryland 3-year Experience," *Journal of Urology* 164 (2000): 1494–1499. E. M. Johnson, J. S. Najarian, and A. J. Matas, "Living Kidney Donation: Donor Risks and Quality of Life," *Clinical Transplantation* 11 (1997): 231–240.

p. 170: *In 2000 Michael M. Abecassis:* M. Abecassis, "Consensus Statement on the Live Organ Donor," *Journal the American Medical Association* 284 (2000): 2919–2926.

p. 171: *Paying for a kidney:* J. Zargooshi, "Iranian Kidney Donors: Motivation and Relations with Recipients," *Journal of Urology* 165 (2001): 386–392.

p. 174: *Klang…and Clyne…measured perceived well-being and functional capacity:* B. Klang and N. Clyne, "Well-being and Functional Ability in Uraemic Patients Before and After Having Started Dialysis Treatment," *Scandinavian Journal of Caring Science* 11 (1997): 159–166.

p. 175: *Mortality on dialysis in two groups of patients:* O. Ifudu, M. Dawood, P. Homel, and E. A. Freidman, "Timing of Initiation of Uremia Therapy and Survival in Patients with Progressive Renal Disease," *American Journal of Nephrology* 18 (1998): 183–198. R. Maiorca, G. Brunori, B. F. Viola, R. Zubani, G. Cancarini, G. Parrinello, and A. De Carli, "Diet or Dialysis in the Elderly? The DODE Study: A Prospective Randomized Multicenter Trial," *Journal of Nephrology* 13 (2000): 267–270.

Glossary

ACTH Adrenocorticotrophic hormone. A hormone secreted by the pituitary gland that stimulates the adrenal cortex to secrete cortisol.

acidosis An acid condition of body fluids. Two types are recognized: (1) metabolic acidosis, in which the concentration of bicarbonate (and therefore the total carbon dioxide [CO_2] level, because bicarbonate is converted to CO_2 before measurement) in the serum is decreased below normal (i.e., is less than 22 mM); this type occurs with great frequency in patients with kidney failure, because the kidneys fail to retain bicarbonate. The resulting acidosis tends to cause protein wasting and may cause fatigue, and should be treated with oral sodium bicarbonate, which is uniformly effective if given in large enough quantities; (2) respiratory acidosis, which is caused by inadequate ventilation (i.e., such as in lung disorders) and is not a feature of kidney failure.

adrenal Two glands, situated on top of the kidneys, that produce important hormones and secrete them into the bloodstream. Each gland is composed of two parts: an outer portion called the adrenal cortex that produces cortisol and aldosterone (among other hormones), and an inner portion called the adrenal medulla that produces epinephrine and norepinephrine.

albumin The predominant protein in plasma or serum. Albumin is synthesized in the liver. A low level of albumin in the plasma may be a sign of malnutrition; it also can be a sign of inflammation. Normal plasma albumin concentration depends to some extent on the method of measurement, unfortunately; according to the Johns Hopkins Hospital Chemistry Laboratory, normal albumin concentration currently is greater than 3.6 g per dl, but this lower limit, as published by the Chemistry Laboratory, has varied over the years.

albuminuria An increase in albumin (see albumin) in the urine.

aldosterone A hormone produced by the adrenal cortex that plays a major role in the regulation of sodium and potassium excretion by the kidneys.

alkalosis An alkaline condition of body fluids. Two types are recognized: (1) metabolic alkalosis, in which the concentration of bicarbonate (and therefore the total carbon dioxide level) in the serum is increased above normal; this type occurs in kidney disease but is almost never a cause of symptoms and can generally be ignored; (2) respiratory alkalosis, in which the concentration of bicarbonate in the serum is reduced.

alpha-blocker One of a group of drugs that block one of the two main pathways of the sympathetic nervous system, which operates without conscious control. Stimulation of the alpha pathways causes blood vessels to constrict, among many other effects. Drugs in this class are used for the treatment of high blood pressure (among other uses).

ALT and AST Two enzymes made in the liver that are also present in traces in the blood; an increase in the levels of these enzymes in the blood is a very sensitive test for liver injury, which is a side effect of statin drugs used to lower serum cholesterol levels.

amino acids Small molecules that constitute the building blocks of protein and are characterized by having an amino group (NH_2) and an acid group (COOH). Proteins are made up of various combinations of 20 different amino acids.

ammonia A small molecule, NH_3, that is very toxic at high levels but is also an important intermediate in the breakdown of protein. It is converted to urea in the liver.

analgesic A kind of drug that lessens pain.

anemia A subnormal level of red cells in blood circulation and therefore of hemoglobin and hematocrit, due to any cause. Normal red cell count is over 4 million per cubic mm of blood. Normal hemoglobin concentration is over 12 g per dl of blood. Normal hematocrit is over 36 percent.

angiotensin A hormone whose precursor, angiotensinogen, is produced by the kidney. It is converted to angiotensin by an enzyme called angiotensin-converting enzyme, found especially in the lungs. Angiotensin has many actions, the most important of which is the constriction of small blood vessels, leading to a rise in blood pressure.

angiotensin-converting enzyme inhibitors (ACEIs) A group of drugs widely used in kidney failure and also in heart failure to reduce blood vessel constriction. They seem to have beneficial effects in both kidney disease and heart disease.

angiotensin receptor blockers (ARBs) A group of drugs that block the angiotensin receptor, thus preventing angiotensin from exerting its blood vessel constricting action. The effects of these drugs are very similar (but not identical) to the effects of ACEIs (see angiotensin-converting enzyme inhibitors).

antidiuretic hormone A hormone secreted into the blood by the pituitary gland that makes the urine concentrated by its effect on the water permeability of the kidney tubules. In the absence of antidiuretic hormone, the urine becomes dilute and its volume increases. The secretion of antidiuretic hormone is stimulated by an increase in osmolality (see osmolality), a reduction of extracellular fluid volume, and also pain or nausea. Its secretion is inhibited by a decrease in osmolality and also by ethanol.

beta-blocker One of a group of drugs that block one of the two main pathways of the sympathetic nervous system, which operates without conscious control. Stimulation of the beta system increases heart rate and the force of contraction of the heart, and dilates certain blood vessels, among many other effects. Drugs in this class are (rather surprisingly) useful in the treatment of high blood pressure and of angina.

blood pressure Contractions of the heart maintain the pressure in the arterial side of the circulation. With each contraction, the pressure rises to a peak (the systolic pressure). Between contractions it levels off at a lower value, maintained by the elastic tension of the arteries and arterioles (the diastolic pressure). It is still not clear whether the adverse consequences of hypertension, in patients with kidney failure, are more closely related to the systolic pressure, the diastolic pressure, or some sort of average of the two, such as the mean arterial pressure (one-third of the systolic plus two-thirds of the diastolic). We used to think that the diastolic was much more important (in patients without kidney failure), but the pendulum has now swung the other way. This may or may not be true of hypertension in kidney disease. So until we learn the answer, it makes sense to try to control both systolic and diastolic blood pressure.

calcium channel blocker One of a group of drugs used in the treatment of hypertension and of angina that act on the conduction of impulses into cells via calcium entry; these actions ameliorate both hypertension and angina.

cholesterol A waxy substance found throughout the body that is an essential component of cell membranes and a precursor of several hormones but is also a factor in the development of arteriosclerosis. The dangerous effects of high cholesterol concentration are well known: Heart attack frequency is directly related to blood cholesterol concentration. Lowering blood cholesterol slows the fatty buildup in the arteries and in some cases can reduce the buildup already there. If you have two or more other risk factors for heart disease or already have heart disease, you have a great deal to gain from lowering your blood cholesterol. These risk factors include cigarette smoking, high blood pressure, diabetes, obesity, physical inactivity, and family history of heart attack at a relatively early age.

The most important fraction of the total serum cholesterol in contributing to heart disease is LDL cholesterol, sometimes known as "bad" cholesterol. LDL cholesterol levels should be less than 130 mg per dl, or ideally less than 100 mg per dl; 130 to 150 is considered borderline, while 160 mg per dl or higher is considered high risk. Another fraction, HDL cholesterol, is known as "good" cholesterol because it seems to prevent heart attacks rather than promote them. Dietary fat increases LDL cholesterol. Exercise and alcohol (in small amounts) increase HDL cholesterol.

clearance The quotient of the rate of excretion divided by the plasma (or serum) concentration.

correlation Clues to possible treatments to slow progression can be obtained from animal experiments or sometimes can be obtained by observing correlations between various measurements and rates of progression (see page 155). A problem arises that often confuses lay readers: a correlation between two variables may suggest cause and effect but does not prove it. Thus if higher values of A are associated with higher values of B, it does not follow that raising B will raise A, or vice versa. Another possibility is that both A and B may be related to an unmeasured quantity, C.

Familiar examples are the endless chain of epidemiological studies of enormous number of patients with a certain disorder, for example, Alzheimer's disease. Let us say that by asking questions the investigators determine that a disproportionate number were nuns. Despite the association being highly significant statistically, cause and effect is unknown. Nevertheless, some readers will infer that chastity does not protect them against Alzheimer's disease.

The only way to ascertain cause and effect for sure is to conduct a prospective, randomized, double-blind trial. "Prospective" means that the trial was planned in advance rather than based on historical records. "Randomized" means that patients were assigned to treatment or placebo by chance, like flipping a coin. "Double-blind" means that neither the patient nor the investigator knows, until the trial ends, whether the subject has been assigned to drug or placebo.

In nutritional studies, blinding is usually impossible, because there is no way the different dietary regimens can be made indistinguishable by the patients. This circumstance casts a shadow on all such trials but is impossible to avoid.

cortisol The main hormone secreted by the adrenal cortex. It plays a major role in the regulation of glucose metabolism and in the metabolism of sodium plus potassium. Cortisol and related hormones (hydrocortisone and prednisone, among many others) also are used as drugs, either to replace deficient production by the adrenal cortex, or, in higher doses, to counteract inflammation in a huge variety of diseases.

creatine A small molecule present mainly in muscle that, when combined with phosphate, is used as a chemical energy storage mechanism. Creatine spontaneously decomposes into the closely related substance creatinine, at a rate that is independent of its location in the body.

creatinine A small molecule derived from the breakdown of creatine and excreted in the urine. It is hardly broken down in the body at all. Because its production tends to be constant, or nearly so, its level in the serum (or plasma) is a rough index of the amount of kidney function present in patients with kidney disease. (The concentrations of creatinine in serum and in plasma are equal.) Normal serum creatinine concentration in men is less than 1.6 mg per dl and in women less than 1.4 mg per dl.

cystoscopy Examination by means of an instrument inserted through the urethra, which permits visualization of the inside of the bladder.

DHEA (dehydroepiandrosterone) A hormone produced in substantial amounts by the adrenal cortex, whose function still remains obscure. It is a precursor to both male and female sex hormones, but otherwise little is known about it, despite much research. It is available without a prescription and is taken by a large number of people for unproven purposes that include improvement of sexual potency, prolongation of life, prevention of cancer, and many others. It is relatively nontoxic.

diabetes A metabolic disorder characterized by abnormally elevated blood levels of glucose. Two distinct types are recognized: insulin-dependent diabetes mellitus (IDDM), in which the production of insulin by the pancreas is inadequate, and noninsulin-dependent diabetes mellitus (NIDDM), in which there is resistance to the action of insulin.

dialysis Generally, exposure of one solution to another across a membrane that permits passage of salts and water but not of large molecules such as protein. In end-stage kidney disease, two kinds of dialysis are employed: In hemodialysis, the blood is circulated through a long coiled tube of permeable material like cellophane that is immersed in a solution containing salts at the desirable physiological concentrations. Urea and creatinine, which accumulate in the blood in renal failure, diffuse out of the blood across the membrane, and thus their accumulation in body fluids is reduced. In peritoneal dialysis, a similar salt solution in injected into the abdomen. The peritoneal membrane permits substances like urea and creatinine to diffuse out of the blood into the salt solution, which is removed after a few hours and discarded; this process is repeated continuously.

diastolic pressure *See* blood pressure.

diuretics Drugs that increase salt excretion by the kidney.

edema An increase in the extracellular fluid volume sufficient to cause palpable swelling of the soft tissues. (This generally requires at least 3 liters of extra fluid, weighing 3 kg or 6.6 pounds.) Edema is detectable at first in the lowest portions of the body, namely the ankles (unless recumbent, in which case it appears on the small of the back). Edema can be detected by pressing with a finger for a few seconds; a "dent" remains (pitting edema).

Epogen and Procrit Commercially produced forms of erythropoietin, a hormone whose synthesis is completed in the kidneys that stimulates the bone marrow to produce red cells. Because in patients with renal disease, the circulating levels of erythropoietin are inadequate to cause the bone marrow to produce enough red cells, anemia often results. (Occult bleeding into the gut is another cause that may need to be ruled out.) Treatment of this condition used to require blood transfusions, but erythropoietin can be administered by intravenous or subcutaneous injection several times a week. They are extremely expensive but highly effective. One problem with their use is that they tend to aggravate hypertension, but only if the dosage is excessive.

equivalent (Eq) A quantity of a substance defined as a number of grams equal to its molecular weight, divided by the number of molecules that enter into reaction with it (typically 1; but for calcium and magnesium, 2).

erythropoietin *See* Epogen and Procrit.

ESRD (end-stage renal disease) As a result of legislation passed in 1972, the federal government supports dialysis and transplantation for patients certified to be at the end stage, in other words, to require dialysis or transplantation (after 30 months). This program now costs many billions, but rehabilitates only a minority of patients.

essential amino acids Amino acids that cannot be made in the body and must therefore be provided in the diet, in amounts sufficient to make up for their continuous breakdown in the body. The essential amino acids in humans are: valine, leucine, isoleucine, phenylalanine, methionine, threonine, histidine, tryptophan, and lysine.

essential hypertension Continuously elevated blood pressure not caused by any known mechanism.

fish oil A product obtained from certain fish, containing a specific kind of fat, that may be useful in the treatment of kidney failure, especially from IgA nephropathy, and may also reduce the incidence of heart attacks.

focal segmental glomerulosclerosis (FSGS) A common type of glomerular disease, frequently characterized by the nephrotic syndrome.

glomerular filtration rate (GFR) The rate at which filtrate of plasma is made in the kidneys. Normal GFR is about 120 ml per min, but considerable variations are seen in normal subjects and also with age and with gender. GFR is the best measure of kidney function in patients with renal disease.

glomerulonephritis A common cause of renal failure, characterized by inflammatory changes in the glomeruli. Many types of glomerulonephritis are recognized.

glomerulosclerosis Scarring of the glomeruli. A common form of glomerular disease.

glomerulus The filter at the start of each kidney unit (the kidney is made up of about 1 million such units) through which blood flows and out of which, into the tubule, flows a filtrate of plasma.

glucocorticoid A hormone from the adrenal cortex (or a synthetic drug of similar structure) that primarily affects glucose metabolism, such as cortisol.

glycosylated hemoglobin A type of hemoglobin formed by the combination of hemoglobin with glucose when hemoglobin is exposed for a prolonged period to elevated blood levels of glucose. It can be measured in the blood to assess the average blood glucose level in preceding weeks. Normally, less than 6.5 percent of circulating hemoglobin is glycosylated. In people with out-of-control diabetes, much higher levels of glycosylated hemoglobin may be seen.

hematocrit The percentage of the volume of whole blood occupied by cells. A low hematocrit (less than 36 percent) means anemia.

hydronephrosis Dilatation of the urine-collecting system within the kidney, associated with thinning of the functional portions caused by chronic obstruction to urinary outflow.

hyperkaliemia High serum (or plasma) potassium concentration.

hypernatremia High serum (or plasma) sodium concentration.

hyperparathyoidism *See* parathyroids.

hypertension Abnormally elevated blood pressure. The upper limit of normal is about 140/90, but probably varies with age.

hypokaliemia Low serum (or plasma) potassium concentration.

hyponatremia Low serum (or plasma) sodium concentration.

IgA Immunogobulin A.

IgA nephropathy A kidney disease caused by abnormalities in IgA.

intercept The calculated value of a function at an x-axis value of zero, obtained by extending the line describing the relationship to the left-hand axis.

interstitial nephritis A type of kidney failure characterized microscopically by signs of chronic inflammation around the tubules. One common cause is problems with urinary drainage in childhood, which lead to chronic infection of the upper urinary tract and eventually to kidney failure. Another common cause is drugs that injure the kidneys, such as lithium.

intravenous pyelogram (IVP) An X ray of the kidneys taken after injection of a dye that is visible on X ray; the outline of the collection system is seen.

ketoacids Chemically synthesized derivatives of amino acids, in which the amino group is replaced with a keto group, that is, an oxygen atom. The ketoacids corresponding to the essential amino acids can, with two exceptions, replace the dietary requirement for the amino acids.

keto analogues Another name for ketoacids (*see* previous entry).

ketoconazole A drug widely used for the treatment of fungus infections. Coincidentally, it has an inhibitory effect on the production of cortisol by the adrenal cortex, as well as a variety of other effects, and slows the progression of kidney failure.

kidney failure The term "chronic kidney failure," like the term "chronic heart failure," is somewhat confusing. It does not mean that the kidneys or the heart has failed. It signifies that the function of the organ is reduced. A better term might be "chronic renal insufficiency," but this is not used as often. The term "chronic kidney disease" includes not only chronic kidney failure but also other chronic diseases of the kidney that are not necessarily associated with renal insufficiency, such as recurrent kidney stones, kidney tumors, chronic infections of the kidney, and the nephrotic syndrome (the combination of excessive loss of protein in the urine, low concentration of protein, especially albumin in the plasma, and accumulation of fluid in the soft tissues). Of these other disorders, only the nephrotic syndrome is considered in this book, because its management and the management of chronic kidney failure have much in common.

left ventricular hypertrophy Enlargement of the wall of the main chamber of the heart, the left ventricle. An early sign of heart disease, often caused by hypertension or by anemia.

lipid An organic compound that has the characteristics of fat. Lipids are poorly soluble in water but are soluble in organic solvents like ether and alcohol, and are greasy to the touch. Examples of lipids found in the body are triglycerides and cholesterol.

loop of Henle A loop present in each kidney unit (nephron) that extends from the outer part of the kidney down toward the center. In the ascending portion of this loop, a large amount of salt is reabsorbed. So-called loop diuretics act here by inhibiting this process.

mean The average of a number of observations.

mean arterial pressure A time-averaged blood pressure calculated as one-third of the systolic pressure plus two-thirds of the diastolic pressure.

median The value above which half of the observations fall and below which the other half fall. The median and the mean of a series of observations may differ considerably if there are a few extremely high or extremely low values. The median is more useful for some purposes.

microalbuminuria An increase in urine protein too small to be detected by the usual clinical tools: specifically, between 30 and 200 mg per day.

mole A quantity of a molecule comprising its molecular weight, in grams.

nephron A unit of the kidney, consisting of a glomerulus and a tubule. The normal kidney contains at least 1 million such units.

nephropathy Kidney disease.

nephrotic syndrome Large amounts of protein in the urine (more than 3.5 g per day), a low level of albumin in the serum (less than 3.5 g per dl), and accumulation of fluid in soft tissues. The nephrotic syndrome usually is accompanied by very high serum levels of cholesterol and triglycerides. Although this definition does not include renal insufficiency, many patients with the nephrotic syndrome eventually develop renal failure. The nephrotic syndrome has many causes, some of which can be diagnosed clinically but many of which require a renal biopsy to diagnose. Conventional treatments include steroids in large dosages, immunosuppressive agents, and ACE inhibitors.

nitrogen balance The difference between nitrogen intake and total nitrogen output. It is a measure of the change in total body protein, which in turn is the best measure of nutrition.

nonsteroidal anti-inflammatory drugs A large groups of drugs that counteract inflammation, but are not chemically related to cortisol (the hormone produced by the adrenal cortex). These include aspirin, acetaminophen (Tylenol), celecoxib (Celebrex), ibuprofen (Advil, Motrin), naproxen (Naprosyn, Aleve), rofecoxib (Vioxx), and many others. All have the potential to cause kidney damage.

nonessential amino acids Amino acids that can be synthesized in the body and are used for protein synthesis. In humans they are: alanine, arginine, aspargine, cystine, glutamine (or glutamate), glycine, proline, serine, and tyrosine.

osmolality The total concentration of all dissolved solids, expressed without regard to their chemical structure. The lab can measure it directly in serum; this is called serum osmolality. This is confusing, because one would suppose that serum sodium concentration reflects the salt content of the body, rather than the ratio of dissolved solids to water. Serum sodium concentration reflects the ratio of dissolved solids to water because sodium salts constitute a major fraction of the total dissolved solids present. Therefore, the concentration of sodium salts (times 2 to include the negatively charged ions like chloride) is nearly the ratio of dissolved solids to water.

oxypurinol A metabolite of allopurinol, produced in the body when allopurinol is administered. Oxypurinol is responsible for allopurinol's therapeutic effect in lowering blood uric acid level and improving the symptoms of gout. Some patients who are allergic to allopurinol may not be allergic to oxypurinol, which therefore might be a preferable drug for them. However, at present it is not marketed in the United States.

parathyroids Four small endocrine glands located near the thyroid gland in the neck, which control plasma calcium concentration, by acting on bone (to stimulate bone reabsorption) and on the kidney tubules (to inhibit phosphate reabsorption, thus increasing phosphate excretion). A fall in plasma calcium concentration or a rise in plasma phosphate concentration stimulates the secretion of parathyroid hormone. In kidney failure, secretion of parathyroid hormone is typically increased and may become excessive. In some cases this condition, secondary hyperparathyroidism, causes severe bone disease when this excessive secretion fails to shut off.

peritoneum The membrane that encloses the intestines and other organs in the abdomen.

plasma Part of the blood; specifically, the clear liquid in which red cells are suspended. To obtain plasma for analysis, it is necessary to add an anticoagulant before centrifugation. (*See also* serum.)

polycystic kidney disease A common cause of kidney failure, attributable to genetic defects and inherited from one parent. Several genetically distinct types are recognized. Cysts, which may reach enormous size, are present in the kidneys. Cysts often are present in the liver too, but usually cause no ill effects. Dilatations of arteries in the brain (aneurysms), however, can cause fatal bleeding. At present, no generally useful treatment is known.

predialysis Refers to renal failure that has not yet become severe enough to require dialysis.

prednisone A synthetic steroid that is widely used in therapy, having effects similar to those of cortisol.

Procrit *See* Epogen.

protein A large molecule comprised of a chain of amino acids.

proteinuria An increase in protein excretion in the urine (usually mostly albumin).

renal tubular acidosis A particularly malignant form of acidosis seen in children, in which the ability of the kidneys to acidify the urine is severely limited. There are several variants. Without treatment, these children fail to grow and develop renal stones and renal failure. Sodium bicarbonate tablets, in substantial dosages (2 to 5 mEq per kg per day), totally correct these problems. If gastrointestinal intolerance becomes a problem, an alternative is the same dosage of Shohl's solution, which contains sodium citrate and citric acid and is reasonably pleasant tasting. Children who need potassium supplementation too may be given Polycitra, which also contains potassium citrate.

salt Sodium chloride.

salt balance The difference between salt intake and salt output in the urine. A positive salt balance means the body is retaining salt; a negative salt balance means the opposite.

serum The liquid remaining after blood has been permitted to clot and the red cells have been removed by centrifugation. Most constituents are measured in serum because it is convenient to obtain. (*See also* plasma.)

sodium polystyrene sulfonate (SPS) An ion exchange resin that can be taken by mouth and releases sodium in exchange for potassium in the intestine. It comes out in the stool. In this way, potassium is removed from the body, and blood potassium concentration falls. It is widely used for the treatment of hyperkaliemia (*see* above).

sonogram An image created by sending ultrasound waves and depicting their reflection.

statins A group of recently discovered drugs that inhibit a specific step in cholesterol synthesis and are very widely used to lower serum cholesterol levels in patients with heart disease but in otherwise normal subjects. Among these are atorvastatin (Lipitor), simvastatin (Zocor), lovastatin (Mevacor), pravastatin (Pravachol), and fluvastatin (Lescol). Their main side effect is liver damage, which is heralded by an increase in serum levels of AST and ALT (*see* above). Another dangerous side effect is muscle damage, which is heralded by muscle pain; if the drug is continued, substances released from the damaged muscle may destroy the kidneys.

steroid One of many substances that have a certain chemical structure and include cholesterol, glucocorticoid hormones, aldosterone, DHEA, and the many forms of vitamin D.

stricture Abnormal narrowing of an interior passageway within a tubular structure, as a vessel or a duct.

systolic pressure *See* blood pressure.

transferrin A protein found in the blood that functions as a carrier for iron and is made in the liver. One of the first signs of protein deficiency is a drop in transferrin concentration.

triglycerides Chemical form in which most body fat is found; specifically, 1 molecule of glycerol is linked to 3 molecules of an organic acid, known as a fatty acid, hence the name "triglycerides."

urea A small molecule containing nitrogen that is produced in the liver and excreted in the urine. It is the main product of the breakdown of protein in the body.

ureter One of two conduits through which urine flows from the kidneys to the bladder.

urethra The conduit through which urine can flow from the bladder to the outside.

vasopressin Another name for antidiuretic hormone.

water balance The difference between intake of water plus all other fluids and water loss, which includes urine volume plus about a quart lost through the skin by evaporation and through the lungs by breathing.

Index